We've all been conditioned to believe that achieving health, leanness and longevity is a difficult, expensive, frustrating and elusive lifelong struggle. It can be, unless you simply give your body what it really needs in the first place.

Lean And Healthy To 100

by
Gordon Filepas

Lean And Healthy To 100

Copyright © 2012 Gordon Filepas
All Rights Reserved

ISBN: 978-0-615-59500-9

Published by Advice For My Children Publications
www.adviceformychildren.com

I dedicate this book to you, my children, because you were my inspiration to create it. You've changed my life for the better in ways you may never know and I cannot imagine going through life without you. I hope this information keeps you and your future families happy, healthy, lean and long-lived.

Love, Dad

Acknowledgements

My goal in researching this information was never to write a book. Once my children suggested it, part of me cringed because I never thought I was a particularly good writer and the thought of doing a "brain dump" of all the relevant information I learned during a 20 year period seemed astonishingly difficult to me. But little by little things began to fall in place, in large part with the help and encouragement of a number of people. First, my wife Kelly who shouldered more than her fair share of what it takes to run a household during the past seven months so that I could organize my thoughts and write in relative peace-and-quiet. Her love, encourage-ment and belief in my ability to complete this project far exceeded my own and powered me through those times when I could have given up. My two wonderful sister-in-laws who, despite their hectic schedules with their own families, made time to review whatever I asked them to so I could obtain their fresh perspective. My editors and creative geniuses Martin and Colin who worked tireless-ly and patiently to meet my deadlines. And to everyone else who helped my family and I through challenging or important times in our lives. Thank you all immensely.

Table of Contents

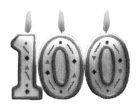

Foreword

After my father and brother both died of cancer just three years apart 20 years ago, I began an impassioned quest to learn the keys to health so my new family would never suffer their fate.

Since then, I've read hundreds of health books, spent thousands of hours researching on the internet, heavily experimented on myself with many different diets, products and supplements trying to figure out the "difference that makes the difference" so getting healthy, lean and long-lived could be achieved easily and inexpensively for my family. I kept the best information I found in a file on my computer called Advice For My Children.

As I began to make sense of things, my family would discuss my findings around the dinner table. Questions from my children would often inspire further research. Then one night my children suggested I write a book about everything they were taught because "Dad, lots of other people could benefit from this information also."

So I began the journey to take all the information I learned from many different sources over the years and compressed it into a single book that contains everything you need and that anyone can understand and benefit from.

I am certain you will be incredibly shocked at how little you need to do to achieve your health goals. There is no "pain" of any kind involved—no dieting, strenuous exercising, special foods, expensive supplements or time consuming rituals. There are no tricks or gimmicks. You just do what is completely natural.

Although you need to do very little, you do need to do something very basic each day. Quite frankly, it's so amazingly easy and inexpensive it's almost laughable.

Once you give your body what it really needs, virtually all of your issues will "self-correct" because that's what your body is designed to do...your weight will normalize, your energy will soar, stress levels will plummet, pain will disappear, you will eat normally, you will sleep better, your hair may return to its natural color, your skin will become tighter, your body will become leaner... all because you are giving your body the absolute foundation of what it needs.

I now believe what natural health experts believe—that 85% or more of the chronic health, weight and aging issues that plague Americans today can be eliminated easily and inexpensively. That's why my family wanted to share this information with everyone.

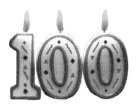

About

We've all been conditioned to believe that achieving health, leanness and longevity is a difficult, expensive, frustrating and elusive lifelong struggle. It can be, unless you simply give your body what it really needs in the first place.

This book is about how to achieve health, leanness, and longevity easily and inexpensively. By longevity, I mean living to at least age 100!

Unlike diet books or programs, this book is not just about losing weight and getting lean. There are plenty of people who have lost a lot of weight who have not necessarily reduced their risk of getting a disease or dying before their time—they just look better. Plenty of thin and lean people get diseases and die young.

There are no guarantees in life. No one knows when they will die. This book is about how to easily and inexpensively stack the odds *heavily* in your favor so that you will live a long, healthy life more easily than you ever thought possible.

I suppose I could have broken this book into three separate books—one about getting healthy, one about getting lean and one about how to live to 100. The reason I included everything in one book is that these three goals can operate independently of each other:

- You can become healthier without becoming lean.

- You can become lean without becoming healthier.

- You can become lean without living longer.

- You can live longer without becoming lean.

- In other words, just because you lose weight doesn't mean you've actually become healthier or will live longer.

Now that you may be thoroughly confused, you'll see what I mean as you start to read through the chapters. My goal in this book is to show you how to achieve all three goals—healthy, lean, longevity—simultaneously by simply giving your a body what it really needs in the first place.

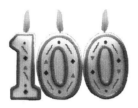

Believe "Time"
Not "Them"

I am going to place a very heavy emphasis throughout this book on common sense. That's because common sense has stood the test of time.

I'm looking at a large maple tree outside my window. A single branch of that tree contains more knowledge about the secrets of the universe and how life works than all the knowledge mankind has discovered since the beginning of time. No amount of human knowledge or technology can identify why the tree does what it does, how it knows what to do each year or how such a large tree can grow from such a tiny seed.

And, we're talking about "just" a tree here—something most of us would agree is only a fraction as complex as the human body. According to *Universe Today*, it's believed that modern humans (homo sapiens) originated about 200,000 years ago in the Middle Paleolithic period in southern Africa. By 70,000 years ago, humans migrated out of Africa and began colonizing the entire planet. They spread to Eurasia and Oceania 40,000 years ago and reached the Americas by 14,500 years ago. One of the oldest sites ever discovered of human settlement is located at Middle Awash in Ethiopia, where humans lived 160,000 years ago.

If you compare the cells in your body to the cells of a human who lived 160,000 years ago, you would learn they all require essentially the same things to remain healthy. For that matter, how to keep human cells healthy isn't really that different from how to keep the cells of an animal or a plant healthy, as you will learn. Modern science appears to mistakenly believe that because technology has increased immensely over the past 100 years while cells have remain unchanged, that alone is reason enough to ignore what cells need and arrogantly believe all cures therefore must come from science and technology. America's healthcare model is based on this premise and it is completely backwards.

For only about 70 years has man eaten commercialized, processed foods and beverages and listened to the voice of the for-profit medical establishment. That means for about 199,930 years man survived by eating naturally and by getting the raw materials his body needed from the Earth. He relied on the innate, natural evolutionary wisdom of his body.

Let's call this commercialized group "Team Them" and our ancestors "Team Time." If you want to stack the odds heavily in your favor and have the best shot at living a long, lean, healthy life easily and inexpensively, which team would you take your advice from:

- Team Time with 199,930 years of experience?

- Team Them with 70 years of experience?

I choose Team Time, how about you? That's why, in this book, I am going to focus heavily on common sense and on the innate evolutionary needs of your body and cells. It's gotten us this far but now it's all being threatened due to our modern ways.

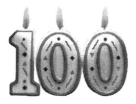

Why I Wrote This Book

About 33 years ago when I was in my teens I went to the doctor for a standard physical and blood work during college. A flu-like virus was going around campus and I was feeling rundown, and I wanted to see if I had acquired it. When my doctor received the lab results he didn't bother sending them—he called my parents immediately. My triglycerides were over 1,100 (normal is less than 150). My cholesterol was over 800 (normal is less than 200). He had never seen triglyceride or cholesterol levels this high in anyone—let alone a teenager—even though he had been in practice many years. My hormones were also severely out of whack and my white blood count was high. He said I was a ticking time bomb and wanted to know what the heck I was doing.

"Nothing" I told him. I thought I was the picture of health. I was lean and muscular, the proper weight for my height with low body fat. I exercised heavily and frequently—jogging about three miles every other day and lifting weights on the days I didn't jog. I was taking a prescription allergy pill daily throughout the year and getting a series of poison ivy shots each spring (I was allergic to poison ivy). My doctor didn't believe any of this was responsible for my condition. He didn't know what to do so he put me on a highly restricted diet of water, lettuce, boiled vegetables and boiled or broiled chicken for almost a year. After about nine months things returned to normal and everything has been normal since. My doctor had no idea how long these imbalances existed because he had never done these tests before.

Fast forward about 12 years.

My father died of cancer in 1991 at the age of 66. My only sibling, a brother, died of cancer three years later at the age of 42. I was at their side most of the year it took them to wither away and die. I clearly remember the moment they each exhaled and did not inhale again.

This was my first experience with real disease or hospitals and it shocked me that all these expensive and advanced medical techniques and highly paid doctors couldn't save them. I mean that was their job—to save people—right? At approximately the same time my wife's grandmother died of cancer and we also experienced two consecutive miscarriages. Our OB/GYN ran a test at the beginning of our third pregnancy that revealed a rare pregnancy condition that caused my wife's blood to thicken, thereby cutting off the blood supply to the fetus. The simple solution was a baby aspirin daily to thin her blood. I was amazed at how something as complex as a miscarriage—with so many potential causes—could be completely prevented by doing something so incredibly simple and inexpensive *right from the start*. We had no problems bearing children from that point forward.

This tsunami of health issues, along with my health issues as a teen, made me wonder about what it really took to keep a body healthy and long-lived. Obviously, simply becoming lean and *looking healthy* was not enough. I wondered what actually causes a disease to start. Why does the body actually die? Why does it all start in the first place? Was it genetics, poisons or toxins, imbalances of some kind, bad luck or just a random occurrence?

Our first child was born about one year after my father died. I *swore* I would never let any of our children suffer the same fate and I wouldn't stop searching until I found the answer. I would learn how to increase their chances of becoming healthy and living longer because simply becoming lean didn't seem to be the answer. I began heavily researching these goals in my spare time. Little did I know that would be the beginning of a 20 year journey of reading hundreds of books, articles, and magazines and spending thousands of hours online trying to figure out what information was real, what truly mattered and then how to piece it all together. I kept my best findings over the years—true kernels of knowledge I wanted to make sure my children knew about—in a file on my computer called "Advice For My Children."

As the information started to make sense we began discussing it around the dinner table as a family. The more we talked about it over the years and the more questions my children asked (kids ask the greatest questions), the more it fueled my research and the more everything came together. Once I started to get a handle on things, I began to relay information to friends and relatives. They were usually quite interested in how I learned about these things and were often very surprised that they had never heard of this information, as they were all very health conscious. My children suggested I write this book because, "Dad, lots of other people could benefit from this information also." That's how this book ultimately came into being.

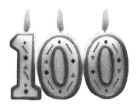

I'm Self Taught
And You Can Be Too

To be clear right from the start, I don't have any fancy or formal health or medical degrees and I am not a medical doctor. I am not a nutritionist or a scientist. I have not taken any correspondence courses on health or wellness. I don't have my own TV, radio or internet show. I'm not a guru of anything as it relates to health or wellness. I am a father of three children; a husband of 24 years; a college graduate; an entrepreneur and a businessman; and most likely, probably a lot like you.

With the internet and all the information that exists in the world today about how to achieve our health goals, anyone who puts in enough "chair time" can become an expert if they are driven to do so. I was driven. There is plenty of great research that's already been done by some very smart and passionate doctors, scientists and natural health experts. The problem I found is that it's scattered everywhere and nowhere could I find everything I wanted in one place.

I'm sure you've heard the saying "80% of your results are achieved by only 20% of your efforts." This 80/20 rule is popular across many different contexts. I believe that 80% of one's health, leanness, and longevity are determined by just 20% of their efforts. I wanted to figure out what the 20% is that produces 80% of the results. I wanted to find the "difference that makes the difference" in the areas of health, leanness, and longevity.

When considering writing this book one of my first questions was "Does the world really need another book on how to get healthy, lean and long-lived?" I never intended to write a book. All my research was done solely for the benefit of my children and my family. They were my one and only target audience. Since this book now exists, obviously my answer to that question was "yes." One of my reasons was because there are thousands of books already on the market about these subjects, yet Americans are still getting sicker and fatter and healthcare costs are still skyrocketing. Clearly, no one in America would complain that there is a shortage of health information, expert opinion or medical technology available today. So, what is the problem? How can a rich nation like America, a nation with access to every scrap of knowledge about how to be healthy, lean and long-lived *not* be healthy, lean and long-lived? Obviously, *something* is missing in America. I'll pinpoint exactly what that appears to be as you read through this book.

Most everything about how to keep us healthy, lean and longer-lived appears to be out of balance. Naturally, I don't want my children to stay on this course. I don't think you want your family or loved ones to either.

I also am not a primary researcher (someone who actually conducts research studies), but rather a secondary researcher (someone who researches the research). Sometimes this is called a meta-researcher. I also experimented pretty heavily on myself to test potential solutions before suggesting them to my family or others.

My primary role in creating this book was simply to be the messenger who pulls all the information and research together into a single source and to explain the information in a way people can understand it. I wanted to convey the information in a way I have not seen before so that it's easily understood by everyone—even someone who knows very little about health.

I believe this book is the only book you and your loved ones will ever need for ultimate health, leanness and longevity. It really is very simple and uncomplicated once you understand the underlying principles of how your body works and what it needs to do the job it's designed to do.

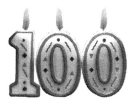

Where I Obtain My Information

I've been researching these subjects for over 20 years for my family and children. The internet did not play a big role in my research until about eight years ago when much more information made its way online. Prior to that most of my information came from books—but not just any books. And certainly not from the books you find at your local national book chain—with the exception of a few. The popular books at your local book store, in my opinion, provide old, tired and recycled information. They put a good-looking, lean person or a doctor on the cover, boast of some incredible result like "Reduce Belly Fat In Three Weeks" or the "Do Nothing Diet" and sit back and wait for the royalty checks to roll in. The books sell, but don't move you any closer to your goals. If you've ever read my blog you'll see numerous frustrating posts about how I visited a book chain, skimmed anywhere from four to eight top selling diet books that night, and experienced the same old recycled information with just bigger claims or better looking, leaner people on the cover. My own teenage children probably know more about how to obtain authentic health, leanness and longevity than many of these authors. The books I read are books you have to dig for and that are off the beaten path. They are usually written by true scientists and researchers, not celebrities or TV personalities. You can now find virtually all of these books online and I list a few of them in the Resources section.

The answers to our health and weight problems lie deeper than just the types of foods you eat, the calories you consume or the ratio of protein, fat and carbohydrates in your diet. A celebrity who rose to fame and fortune from a reality TV show and who now has a bestselling diet book can't compete with the innate wisdom in each of your cells that has been tested, refined and retested during the past 200,000 years of human life on Earth. Anyone can work out five hours a day and get lean. Most people can't and don't want to do that.

I believe the contents of this book represent the absolute easiest and least expensive, common sense way to get healthy, lean and long-lived. You will achieve all three goals simultaneously with no extra effort.

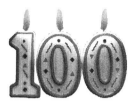

Test Your Knowledge About Health, Leanness And Longevity

Losing weight, getting healthy, lean, energetic, and youthful has taken on a circus-like atmosphere in America. It's a multibillion dollar a year industry that really doesn't need to exist. We've all been conditioned to believe that achieving these goals is difficult, frustrating, expensive, complicated and a lifelong struggle. But, it's truly easy and inexpensive—once you understand how your body works. In a perfect world we would learn all the answers to the following questions in middle school and high school and virtually eliminate health and weight issues in our country. Unfortunately, the way America's healthcare system is currently set up puts the burden on the individual citizen to figure out what works and what doesn't.

See how many of these questions you can answer:

1. How long is the human body capable of living to in good health?

2. Where does America rank on longevity compared to other countries?

3. What's the single most important thing you can do to fix your metabolism and get it burning as hot as possible without doing any exercise?

4. How do America's healthcare costs and outcomes compare to other countries?

5. How can countries where people don't have any modern healthcare, medicine or technology—and who rarely exercise—live longer than Americans?

6. How can the Japanese smoke many more cigarettes than Americans yet have fewer cases of lung cancer and the longest average lifespan of any country?

7. How long can a human cell live if cared for properly?

8. How can the French drink more alcohol and eat much more fat than Americans and have fewer cases of heart disease?

9. If high cholesterol is bad and supposedly causes heart attacks, why do about half of the people who have heart attacks have below normal cholesterol?

10. How many nutrients does the human body need every day to remain healthy, according to natural health experts?

11. How many disease states do natural health

experts estimate you can reduce or eliminate by getting these nutrients?

12. Most people who die of natural causes die of what?

13. Why do you get tired, sick, fat, age and die?

14. You can receive all your nutrients from a very healthy, natural and organic diet or from the diet outlined in the food pyramind, right?

15. Why does someone else's body shed fat while your body stores fat, all things being equal?

16. What's the single most important step you can take to make your body not want to over-eat? (hint - it's not fiber or water).

17. If you can only afford to supplement from one category of these nutrients which should it be and why?

18. If you have regular bowel movements you don't need to worry about toxic buildup in your body, right?

19. Three bowel movements a week is fine, right?

20. If you' want to detoxify which methods work best?

21. Farmers receive all kinds of subsidies from the government for different things. How much do they receive in subsidies for growing foods that contain more nutrients?

22. If you receive lots of electrolytes, herbs, or antioxidants from popular sports drinks that's good, right?

23. Drinking lots of water every day is very healthy, right?

24. You should drink at least two eight ounce

glasses of fluids with each meal, right?

25. What is the primary cause of cravings?

26. Do you know the most common sense way to stop cravings?

27. What actually causes hunger?

28. When you're hungry what's your body actually asking for?

29. Why does your body remain hungry even after you've just eaten?

30. Are overeating and obesity conditions of excess or deficiency? Why?

31. Should you count calories and fat, protein and carbohydrate grams? Why or why not?

32. When you are trying to decide what to eat at mealtime or as a snack, what are the things you should think about?

33. What is the major difference between the needs of human cells today vs. those of our ancestors from 100,000 years ago?

34. What is healthier—a high protein, high fat, or high carbohydrate meal?

35. The best way to lose weight is to eat less and exercise more, right?

36. Which fats should be avoided and why?

37. What makes some fats dangerous?

38. Which carbohydrates should be avoided and why?

39. If you want to reduce stress and cope better what nutrients can help?

40. How can you help your children behave better even if they are exhibiting hyperactive, compulsive, defiant, addictive, destructive or

hyperactive behaviors?

41. If you want to sleep better and have more energy what should you do?

42. When you hear the results of a new health study you should follow that advice, right?

43. Exotic nutrients from jungles, fruits, herbs, supplements, juices or extracts are the real secret to health and longevity, right?

44. What types of foods should you eat every day?

45. What ratio of protein, fats and carbohydrates should you eat?

46. Just because someone loses weight and reaches their ideal weight, does that mean they will live longer than you or have a lower risk of getting a disease? Why or why not?

47. If someone is skinny, lean or "ripped" does that mean they have a lower risk of dying or getting diseases?

48. Eating four to seven small meals a day is better than eating three normal size meals a day, right?

49. You should never eat after 7 p.m. because you'll gain weight, right?

50. Breakfast should be your biggest meal of the day, right?

51. If someone exercises regularly does that mean they will live longer than you or is at a lower risk of getting a disease?

52. If your goal is to look, feel and perform your best at any age what are the top things you need to do?

53. How many calories do you need to maintain

your weight or to lose weight?

54. What is the absolute easiest and least expensive thing you can do to improve your health, achieve your ideal weight and live as long as possible, even if you are the world's laziest person?

55. What is the number one thing America's food and beverage makers can do to improve the health of Americans and improve their sales and profits?

56. Eliminating childhood obesity is difficult, right?

57. What's better for your health—lifting weights or cardiovascular exercises?

58. What percentage of how you look, feel, and perform is determined by what you eat?

59. Your biggest calorie burn during the day comes from exercise, right?

60. A typical human body typically contains less than 50 different toxins, right?

61. The first thing you should do when you're hungry is breathe deeply, right?

62. Our healthcare system is rewarded for making us live longer, healthier lives, right?

63. Why don't physically fit people like athletes or very lean people like bodybuilders live as long, on average, as couch potatoes?

64. Why do 85% of people using diet programs gain back all the weight they lost and then some?

This is a long list for sure, but very important to know. You will learn the answers to these questions and others by the time you finish this book.

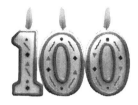

Why We Get Fat, Sick, Age And Die

The reason I bring this up here, early on, is because I want you to start thinking about your health and weight problems in a different way so as you read through this book, light bulbs may start going off in your head. I will go into detail to answer this topic later, but for now, I want you to understand that you get fat, sick, age and die from an imbalance in your body. The imbalance begins due to one of only two simple reasons, as you will learn. This imbalance creates a cascade of additional imbalances—like dominos falling. As the imbalances increase you get fatter, sicker and age faster until the imbalances overtake your body's ability to fight back. Then you die. You die from an imbalance—but of what? That's what the remainder of the book is about.

Your body can live much longer than you think. You will learn that your body should be able to live in good health to age 120—140 and quite a few people have lived even longer than this, up to age 145. Many experts believe that living to 120 should be the new norm (rather than to 78) because the human cell is considered by some experts to be immortal if given the raw materials and environment it needs.

Keep in mind your body is the most amazing machine on the planet. It is completely dynamic and adaptive—always doing its best to keep you alive and healthy regardless of what you do to it. Your body never "turns" on you. It is always trying to rebuild itself to become as strong as possible. Unfortunately, our human choices and the toxins in our environment can easily override our body's ability to manage what's happening to it. The imbalances persist and result in our gaining weight, becoming sick, aging and ultimately dying.

In simple terms, your body is just a bunch of cells—about 100 trillion of them. In each cell is DNA. The DNA controls everything in each cell. As long as the conditions are right for that DNA to replicate normally and without incident, you will look and feel great. You will age wonderfully. You will be in great health. But, as you make poor choices; as your body doesn't receive the raw materials it needs; as toxins invade your cells—the DNA cannot fully "switch on" because it doesn't have the raw materials it needs to do so.

Imagine your DNA as a dimmer switch that controls the brightness of a lamp in your home. When the dimmer switch is fully switched on the light is as bright as it can be. But what if the dimmer switch could only turn halfway on due to a malfunction of some type? No matter how hard you tried to push that switch all the way up, it would never move beyond halfway. The lights remain dim. That's where most of America is today—with the DNA switch only halfway on. Their "lights" are dim. The malfunction I refer to is really an imbalance. Correct the imbalance and the DNA switch will turn fully on.

Some experts believe that the fraying of the ends of the DNA strand is the cause of aging. These ends are called telomeres and they are often compared to the little plastic pieces that encase the end of your shoelaces. Their theory is that once these ends become frayed the DNA cannot replicate properly and therefore can't fully switch on to do its job. The fraying of telomeres may be a factual phenomenon, but I chalk it up as just another sign of aging due to imbalances in your body. There's no reason for the end of your DNA to fray if your body is receiving all the raw materials it needs and is able to rebuild itself faster than it breaks down.

Fortunately, imbalances are easy and inexpensive to fix. I cannot guarantee 100% success of course however, the information in this book will allow you to heavily—and I really mean heavily—stack the odds in your favor that you will lead a long, healthy, lean life as easily, inexpensively and naturally as possible.

Also remember, you don't get fat, sick, age or die from a *lack of* pharmaceuticals, radiation, chemotherapy, stem cells or medical technology. You get fat, sick, age and die because you're not giving your body what it needs in the first place so your body naturally breaks down. It's not rocket-science, it's just common sense.

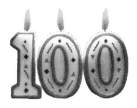

The Role Of Genetics

The DNA characteristics passed to you from your ancestors are called your genes. They determine things like your height, shape of your body frame, eye color, hair color, skin tone and many other physical factors and characteristics about you. As they relate to health, your genes can also determine things like your predisposition to various health conditions like eczema, allergies, propensity to develop a disease, etc. Western medicine makes the error of putting too much emphasis on your genetics rather than on other factors like nutrition and lifestyle choices. This goes hand in hand with America's disease treatment model (rather than disease prevention model) that suggests there's very little you can do to solve your problem (due to your genes), so take this medicine and simply treat your symptoms forever. You were dealt a bad genetic hand in life so just make the best of it.

In reality, your genes determine the path you *might* take, not the path you *will* take. You have a lot of control over the path you take in life. If your ancestors had heart disease, for example, you may have a greater chance of acquiring heart disease than me. But, it does not mean you will get heart disease. It means if you do what your ancestors did you will probably get heart disease. But, you can change your ways and never suffer that fate.

I remember hearing two doctors arguing on a TV show about the role of genetics. Doctor #1 was a naturopath and said that genetics have very little to do with health outcomes. Doctor #2 was a traditionally trained Western physician who indicated that genetics were the overriding factor that determined health outcomes. Doctor #2 pointed to a healthy country like Japan and said something to the effect of "those people have good genes and they stay healthy." Doctor #1 indicated that if you take a "genetically superior" Japanese baby and a "genetically inferior" American baby from an overweight family, and switched them at birth so each is raised by the other culture, the genetically superior Japanese baby will suffer American diseases and the genetically inferior American baby will grow to be healthy, strong and long-lived. In other words, Doctor #1 was saying your health and longevity are determined much more by your lifestyle choices than by your genes. You can easily make the unhealthy healthy and the healthy unhealthy simply by your choices.

There are two books you should read that prove the point I made above. *Nutrition And Physical Degeneration* by Dr. Weston A. Price is the first. He showed that extremely healthy cultures around the world could literally change the health of their offspring in just one generation simply through food, nutrition and lifestyle choices. The second is *Pottenger's Cats: A Study In Nutrition* by Francis Marion Pottenger. He showed how cats can quickly change their genetic propensity to debilitating conditions and diseased offspring in just a single generation simply by changing their diet.

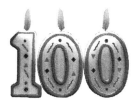

Losing Weight Is The Primary Problem To Solve, Right?

Most people are very good at losing weight. Some people are even true experts at it. The problem is keeping the weight off. The latest statistic I heard is that over 85% of people gain back all the weight they've lost within five years. Many gain back even more weight than they lost. Losing weight is where the focus of most diet and weight loss programs begins and ends in America. Problem is, the weight itself is not the root cause of the problem— it's only the symptom of the problem. Unless you eliminate the root cause of overeating the weight will just keep coming back. That's great for the diet industry but bad for you.

The current focus in America of simply losing weight is a top down approach. To lose weight you simply eat less and exercise more. It's all about calories in minus calories out. There is virtually no focus on correcting the imbalance within the body that *causes* the symptom or side-effect of excess weight in the first place. The root imbalance lies far deeper in the body at the cellular and DNA level. Fix the root cause of the imbalance and just about everything resulting from the imbalance automatically fixes itself, including ill health and excess weight. This approach—first giving your body the spectrum of raw materials it needs—is a bottom up approach.

How many of you reading this book are overweight or unhealthy because someone else stuffs food in your mouth all day? Raise your hand please. If someone ties you up and force-feeds you against your will hold that hand up high! I hope no one raised their hand. You're overweight or unhealthy because *you* are choosing to put the wrong things in your mouth. So, why are *you* doing that? *Something* is disrupting your ability to eat naturally. It could be a physical issue or an emotional issue. The good news is that both of these are easy to fix, as you will learn in an upcoming chapter.

I recently spoke with two plus size women who were sitting at a table near me at a restaurant. I overheard them complaining how they would gain 20 pounds and then lose 20 pounds and they appeared distressed over this issue. I introduced myself and mentioned I was writing a book about this subject and inquired if they would mind if I asked them a question. They agreed, so I asked them if they knew how many nutrients experts say the human body needs each day to remain healthy and lean easily and inexpensively? They looked at each other and shrugged their shoulders and said collectively "We have no idea." They said they had just come from their weekly meeting at one of America's most popular weight loss companies. Here they are—spending their hard-earned money at one of America's top weight loss companies and they don't know the nutritional raw materials they need to lose weight easily and effortlessly? Shouldn't that have been one of the very *first* things they were taught if the goal was to really keep the weight off?

America's emphasis on simply losing weight, exercising more and eating healthier doesn't solve the _real_ root problem and may actually promote more disease and a shorter life. Do people who are lean or at their ideal weight still get cancer, strokes, heart disease, diabetes, Alzheimer's, Parkinsons, kidney disease or virtually any other known disease? Of course they do. That's why simply losing weight, eating healthy and exercising are not good indicators of how healthy you are, how long you will live or whether or not you will acquire a chronic or life threatening disease.

This book will provide you the clarity required to know exactly what to do so you can take responsibility for your own health and weight issues.

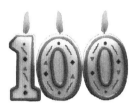

Common Qualities Of The World's Healthiest And Longest Living People

Remember I stated earlier that we were going to put a lot of value on common sense in this book? A common sense starting point might be to look around the world to learn why certain areas have so many people that reach the age of 100. We simply want to copy what those people do. Quite a bit of attention has been focused on the world's healthiest and longest living people in the past. Their bodies are just like ours, right? So what works for them will work for us. We simply need to observe and understand what these people do—and do it.

I'm not going to go into all the details of what these cultures do because there are already entire books dedicated to that subject. Here are just a few of them:

- *Nutrition and Physical Degeneration* by Dr. Weston A. Price.

- *Blue Zones* by Dan Buettner

- *Immortality* by Dr. Joel Wallach

Generally, the cultures with the greatest longevity have these common elements:

- A low calorie diet of less than 2,000 calories per day. This is often referred to as a calorie-restricted diet. (This type of diet also puts very little stress on their digestive system and you will learn why that's important in a future chapter.)

- A diet that's very nutrient-dense and rich in the complete spectrum of required nutrients.

- A focus on whole unprocessed foods, fats and oils including fruits, vegetables, nuts, seeds, beans and grains. Meat, if eaten, is typically consumed sparingly—like a side dish.

- Food is eaten both cooked and raw (raw means cooking temperature does not exceed approximately 118 degrees Fahrenheit).

- They often consume some fermented foods for intestinal health.

- They consume few if any toxins or pollutants from the air, water, beverages, foods or medicines.

- They have a strong sense of purpose and reason to wake up every day and it's more than just to "make money." Their purpose is the work they do and a feeling they are making a difference, no matter how small. A long workday is also very common and they often work six days each week.

- They help and support each other and have a strong social network.

- Most drink some type of alcoholic beverage regularly and in moderation.

- They do virtually no separate form of exercise as their basic daily activities appear to provide enough movement.

- Their cooking methods are traditional, not high tech (e.g. no microwave ovens).

- They take personal responsibility for their own health.

It's fascinating to me how these cultures remain so healthy and disease free with no modern medicines or medical technology. They just do the basics and that simplicity is the genius behind their success. Notice that they are not eating any fat burners, bizarre super foods, crazy food combinations or any rare, exotic or secret discoveries. Likewise, these cultures typically do not use any toothpaste, toothbrushes, mouthwashes, dental floss or other dental cleaning devices yet they commonly have perfectly healthy, sparkling white teeth without cavities or the need for orthodontic appliances. It's truly astonishing. You can only attribute this to their diet and to the nutrients they receive. They're really just doing the basics. We're going to adopt the same model but we will have to do things a little differently to compensate for the numerous problems our modern society has created.

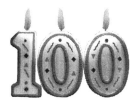

Top 15 Causes
Of Death In America

Not to be morbid, but I think it's important to start with the end in mind to set the stage for the remainder of this book. Let's see what people in America are ultimately dying from so we can learn from their mistakes and perhaps eliminate what's causing these deaths in the first place.

Below are the top 15 causes of death in America based on the most recent data available on www.worldlifeex-pectancy.com. This data comes from the World Health Organization, states and other public resources. For all the good things that can be said about living in America, eating healthy food and making healthy lifestyle choices isn't one of them. You can assume that you will contract one or more of the following ailments if you don't follow the suggestions contained in this book. I show three additional numbers for each cause of death—the state where this cause of death ranks highest per 100,000 people, the state where this form of death ranks lowest per 100,000 people and the average number of deaths from this cause across America per 100,000 people.

Our goal is to greatly reduce or eliminate your chance of death from as many of these causes as possible.

Death Rate Per 100,000

Rank	Cause of Death	State with the highest death rate from this cause	Average number of deaths from this cause	State with the lowest death rate from this cause
1	Heart Disease	Mississippi (265)	190	Minnesota (130)
2	Cancer	Kentucky (213)	178	Utah (127)
3	Stroke	Arkansas (57)	42	New York (28)
4	Chronic Lung Disease	Oklahoma (61)	41	Hawaii (19)
5	Accidents	New Mexico (67)	40	New York (25)
6	Alzheimer's	Washington (41)	23	New York (9)
7	Diabetes	West Virginia (36)	23	Nevada (13)
8	Influenza & Pneumonia	Tennessee (22)	16	Florida (9)
9	Nephritis/ Kidney Disease	Louisiana (26)	15	North Dakota (6)
10	Blood Poisoning	Louisiana (20)	11	California (3)
11	Suicide	Alaska (22)	11	D.C (6)
12	Liver Disease	New Mexico (18)	9	New York (6)
13	Hypertension/Renal	Mississippi (14)	7	Alaska (4)
14	Parkinson's Disease	Utah (8)	6	D.C. (4)
15	Homicide	D.C. (24)	6	New Hampshire (1)

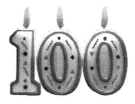

How Long You Can Live

Now that we know what most Americans will die from, let's learn how long different segments of our population live on average.

Health experts estimate the human body is capable of living to between 120-140 years of age in good health. Today, the average lifespan in America is 78.2 years according to the World Health Organization public data for the year 2010 on the website www.worldlifeexpectancy.com. America ranks 29th in life expectancy out of 192 countries. Japan has the longest life expectancy at 82.2 years.

Additionally, this site reports on something called Healthy Life Expectancy. It measures the years of your life that are free of disability and other impairments. For example, although Americans have an average life expectancy of 78.2 years their Healthy Life Expectancy is only 70 years, making America 34th out of 192 countries. That means Americans can expect to live *with* debilitating conditions for eight years on average or about 10% of their lives. Japan has a Healthy Life Expectancy of 76 years. The following summary table, part of which was obtained from Nationmaster.com, reveals that Japan spends less than half of what America spends on healthcare yet outlives us and avoids our obesity problems, while also having 50% more people reach age 100:

	America	Japan
Life Expectancy	78.2 years	82.2 years
Rank	29th	1st
Healthy Life Expectancy	70 years	76 years
Rank	34th	1st
Healthcare spending/person	$7,250	$2,750
Rank	1st	20th
Percentage of population obese	30.6%	3.2%

It's also enlightening to compare the average lifespan of various groups in America:

- The average American lives to 78.2 years of age. This includes couch potatoes as well as health nuts. (LESSON: Everything we are doing or not doing is allowing us to reach about 61% of our optimal lifespan.)

- American physicians. According to Kevin Kenward of the American Medical Association, "Based on over 210,000 records of deceased physicians, our data indicate the average lifespan of a physician is 70.8 years." Doctors typically die from diabetes, cancer, stroke and heart disease...the same things we go to them to fix and prevent and they die on average eight years earlier than the average couch potato. (LESSON: Knowing a lot about Western medicine, treating disease and having the world's most advanced medical technology does little to increase health or lifespan.)

- Professional athletes live on average to 67 years of age and NFL players to 58 years of age according to Strengthplanet.com. No professional athlete in the past 80 years has ever lived to 100 years of age. (LESSON: Being physically fit, exercising a lot and getting lean does not guarantee health or a long life span.)

- Vegetarians seem to reach age 100 at about the same rate as non-vegetarians, which is infrequent. Albert Einstein, a vegetarian, died at age 76. (LESSON: The sole act of being a vegetarian, which has the benefit of reducing digestive stress on the body, still does not guarantee a long life.)

- No Nobel Prize winner has ever lived to 100 years of age. The average lifespan for the nominees (including winners) was 76 years. (LESSON: Being a genius or very smart does not guarantee health or a long lifespan.)

- No billionaire has ever lived to 100 years of age. The average lifespan of a billionaire is 66 years of age according to a study by Forbes magazine, March 2011. (LESSON: Money can't buy health or longevity. People from the poorest countries of the world live longer, on average, than billionaires.)

- No body builder has ever lived to 100. (LESSON: Being super lean, muscular, "ripped" and exercising a lot does not guarantee health or a long lifespan.)

So if the choices of these groups don't make them live longer, then what does? That's the million dollar question. You will learn the answer later in this book.

Remember that, on average, your heart will stop beating at approximately age 78 if you live in America. And, you will probably die from one of the top 15 causes listed in the previous chapter. All the things you've eaten in your lifetime, drank, smoked, done, worried about, stressed over, enjoyed—plus all the medicines you've taken, plus all the medical technology you've had access to only gets you a lifespan of 78.2 years, on average. That doesn't sound very compelling to me if our human potential is 120-140 years. 78 years is about a 35% shorter lifespan than 120 years or only 61% of your potential!

There must be *something else* we're missing in America...

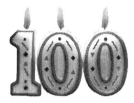

What's Our Healthcare System Doing About It?

Most people realize that America's healthcare system is on an unsustainable course. Some believe it's a bubble that's ready to pop, just like the technology bubble that popped in the year 2000 and the housing bubble that popped in 2008. Bubbles exist because the trajectory of an industry can't be sustained in the future. What's happening isn't real or ecological. The foundation of the industry is based on misinformation, confusion, deceit or greed. The value for things has been falsely inflated. You don't know what's real or unreal—like trying to find your way out of the hall of mirrors at a carnival fun house. Bubbles are wake-up calls, reality checks. Whatever misinformation is fueling the bubble is ultimately exposed. Then, the bubble pops and everything readjusts to normal, realistic and sustainable levels.

If America's healthcare system was a corporation, it would have gone out of business a long time ago. Why? Because what corporation can allow costs to spiral out of control while producing so few tangible results? It's like an investment firm endlessly investing money in a company that makes a terrible product that's also the most expensive product in its industry. It defies common sense and is completely unrealistic. Yet, that's what's happening in America. America is throwing much more money at healthcare than any country in the world, yet producing inferior results.

Please recall the table from the previous chapter that shows Japan, the longest-lived country in the world, spends only half of what America spends on healthcare, yet lives longer than us and doesn't suffer from our obesity problems.

Below is brief glimpse into America's healthcare system today and it's not pretty:

- Child obesity rates are increasing. According to the National Institutes Of Health (NIH), in the past 30 years, the prevalence of childhood obesity has more than doubled among children ages two to five, has tripled among youth ages six to 11, and has more than tripled among adolescents ages 12 to 19.

  - Schools are adding to the problem. An article in *Men's Health* magazine November 2008 titled "Why Are Schools Selling Junk Food To Kids?" discusses in detail why this is happening. The schools need money. Campus vending machines and cafeterias are filled with the foods that make students fat. The trouble is, the money they bring in is too good for schools to pass up because it helps offset decreased government funding.

- Adult obesity is at an all time high with over two-thirds of the population being overweight and 30% considered obese, according to the NIH.

- Health insurance premiums have nearly doubled since 2000—a rate of increase that's three times faster than wage increases (www.kff.org).

- Life expectancy in the U.S. is 29th in the world, below most developed nations and some developing nations. It is below the average life expectancy for the European Union.

- The World Health Organization in 2000 ranked the U.S. healthcare system as the highest in cost, first in responsiveness, 37th in overall performance, and 72nd by overall level of health (among 191 member nations included in the study).

- The Commonwealth Fund ranked the United States last in the quality of healthcare among similar countries and notes U.S. care costs the most. (Wikipedia.com, U.S. Healthcare System).

- According to the Employee Benefits Research Institute, one of the biggest drains on boomer retirement savings will be healthcare costs. Medicare pays for just over half of the healthcare expenses that the typical elderly person will face, estimates EBRI. A couple who is 65 today will need nearly $300,000 to cover those costs. EBRI also states that nearly half of early boomers, born between 1948 and 1954, and 44% of late boomers, born between 1955 and 1964, may not be able to afford even basic living expenses in retirement.

- An often cited study by Harvard Medical School

and the Canadian Institute for Health Information determined that some 31% of U.S. healthcare dollars, or more than $1,000 per person per year, went to healthcare administrative costs, nearly double the administrative overhead in Canada on a percentage basis.

- A report by the U.S. Surgeon General found that mental illnesses are the second leading cause of disability in the nation and affect 20% of all Americans. It is estimated that less than half of all people with mental illnesses receive treatment due to factors such as stigma and lack of access to care.

- According to *Health Affairs*, $7,498 was spent on every woman, man and child in the United States in 2007, representing 20 percent of all national spending. Costs are projected to nearly double to $12,782 per person by 2016.

- Half of all bankruptcies in America are caused by medical bills.

- America represents about five percent of the world's population but consumes almost half of the world's prescription medicines. In 2006 that totalled close to $289 billion in prescription drug use, followed by the European Union and Japan (Mercola.com).

- In 2001, 84.6 percent of all substances implicated in fatal poisonings were pharmaceutical drugs, according to that year's American Association of Poison Control Centers (AAPCC) report.

- According to the Agency For Healthcare Research and Quality, our healthcare system lacks safety controls that endanger frontline workers and patients. Staffing levels are dangerously low in hospitals, nursing homes and other healthcare facilities. As a result medical errors are rising—and account for an estimated 44,000 to 98,000 needless deaths each year.

- The Kaiser Family Foundation (www.kff.org) issued a report in 2010 stating that the average number of prescriptions per person in the U.S. rose from 10.2 in 1999 to 12.6 in 2009.

- According to PRIME Institute for Families USA, the average number of prescriptions per senior citizen in 2010 was a staggering 38.5.

- The Kaiser report stated that in 2008, name brand drugs averaged $137.90 per prescription—almost four times the $35.22 cost of generic drugs.

- The Journal of the American Medical Association (JAMA) reported that while 10,000 people die annually from illegal drug use, an estimated 106,000 (an average of 290 each day) hospitalized patients die each year from properly prescribed and administered drugs, while 2,000,000 more suffer serious side effects (an average of 5,479 each day).

- Below is how doctor's office visits broke down for 2006 data (Center For Disease Control (CDC), August 6, 2008 study press release):

  - In 2006 Americans made 1.1 billion visits to doctors' offices, emergency rooms and outpatient facilities. That's a 26% increase since 1996.

- The most frequent visits were for babies under age one (9.4 visits per year) and those over age 65 (7.4 visits a year).

- Least likely to see a doctor were ages five to 14 years old (2.3 times a year).

- Prescriptions were handed out in seven out of every 10 visits, totalling 2.6 billion prescriptions for medications in 2006.

  - The most often prescribed medications were pain killers (319,958), cholesterol medications (112,430), antidepressants (97,812), sedatives and hypnotics (84,627) and anti-diabetic drugs (81,926).

- Emergency room visits soared 32% between 1996 and 2006.

- The responsiveness of America's health-care system ranks 37th of 190 countries but spending per person ranks first (http:// en.wikipedia.org/wiki/WHO's ranking of health care systems).

- In terms of health care spending per person, America ranks first, spending 50% more per person than the number two country, Norway. Japan, the longest lived and healthiest country in the world, ranks 20th in health care spending per person (http://www.ask. com/wiki/List of countries by total health expenditure (PPP) per capita).

- One of my favorite charts is on the following page. It shows the cost per person for health-care of numerous countries compared to each other and to themselves. Of course the highest cost per person comes from America by a large margin. It is interesting to note that each country's healthcare costs doubled or nearly doubled in just a 12 year period! This is completely unsustainable.

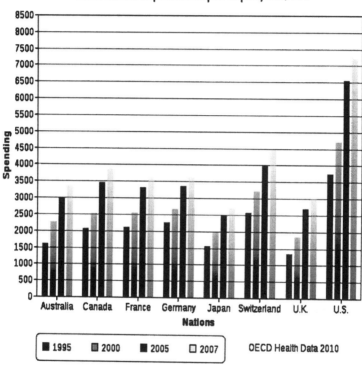

Total health expenditure per capita, US$ PPP

- I would urge everyone to read the article at http://www.kaiseredu.org/Issue-Modules/US-Health-Care-Costs/Background-Brief.aspx. It provides many valuable statistics and openly discusses what is contributing to skyrocketing healthcare costs as well as possible solutions. Prevention is mentioned as only a minor part of the plan, which is unfortunate. The article also contains a pie chart that shows how our healthcare dollars are spent. Seventy-five percent (75%) of the total cost of healthcare is for the treatment of chronic diseases, the same diseases natural health experts believe can be eliminated by simply giving your body the basic raw materials it needs so it can do its job properly ("U.S. Health Care Costs", KaiserEDU.org, available at http://www.kaiseredu.org/Issue-Modules/US-Health-Care-Costs/Background-Brief.aspx, The Henry J. Kaiser Family Foundation, 2011).

- In 2011 the average healthy working American spent over $4,100 on health insurance premiums per year. Employers spend almost $11,000. That's over $15,000 per year for your health insurance premiums ("Average Annual Health Insurance Premiums and Worker Contributions for Family Coverage, 2009-2011", Kaiser Fast Facts, available at http://facts.kff.org/ chart.aspx?ch=2268, The Henry J. Kaiser Family Foundation, 2011).

- Health insurance premiums are expected to increase over the next eight years by between 80% -100% ("Projected Health Insurance Premiums for Family Coverage, Assuming Average Growth Rates, from 1999-2009 and 2004-1999", Kaiser Fast Facts, available at http://facts.kff.org/ chart.aspx?ch=1188, The Henry J. Kaiser Family Foundation, 2011).

- Healthcare costs are skyrocketing much faster than inflation or employee wage increases. The Kaiser Foundation notes, "Premiums for employer-provided health insurance, where 150 million Americans get their coverage, jumped 9% in 2011 while workers' wages grew just 2%, according to our annual employer survey. The average family policy now costs more than $15,000 per year, more than the cost of a Chevy Aveo or a Ford Fiesta. Since we began doing this survey thirteen years ago, worker contributions to premiums have increased 168%, wages 50%, and inflation 38%" ("Cumulative Increases in Health Insurance Premiums, Workers' Contributions to Premiums, Inflation, and Workers' Earnings, 1999-2011", Kaiser Fast Facts, available at http://facts.kff.org/chart.aspx?ch=2280, The Henry J. Kaiser Family Foundation, 2011).

Of course I could go on forever providing charts, articles, and commentaries like those above showing how out of control our healthcare system is, but I'm sure by now you get the point.

Unfortunately, America's healthcare system is currently designed to create dependency and maximize revenue for the companies involved. There is little incentive to prevent disease in the first place or to get the word out to all Americans about how to do this. How can diabetes organizations say diabetes is incurable when doctors are curing it in less than 30 days using only food (http://www.youtube.com/watch?v=ZZe-igIE4dI&feature=related)? How can cancer organizations spend billions of dollars over the past 60 years "investing" in cancer cures and still not produce a cure...when medical doctor and Ph.D. Otto Warburg, back in 1931, routinely gave animals cancer and then cured them and won a Nobel Prize for it? (See his paper: *The Prime Cause and Prevention of Cancer*, Dr. Otto Warburg Lecture delivered to Nobel Laureates on June 30, 1966 at Lindau, Lake Constance, Germany. You can also link to a New York Times article here http://www.athenstalks.

com/nobel-laureate-dr-otto-warburg-md-phd-makes-ny-times). When you hear various organizations in America trumpet that there are no cures for many diseases, in most cases that doesn't mean there are really no cures – it means there are no "patentable" cures created by man that can lock in profits for many years to come. Supposedly the top 10 pharmaceutical companies in the Fortune 500 generate more profit than the other 490 companies do combined, so their approach is obviously working (for them). America's emergency and trauma care system is the best in the world and no one would argue that. However, when it comes to preventing diseases in the first place and teaching people about prevention, "fuggeddaboutit". Perhaps that's why physicians have been dropping out of the America Medical Association (AMA) where now only an estimated 15% of the physicians in America even belong to the AMA (http://www.ncbi.nlm.nih.gov/pmc/articles/PMC3153537/?tool=pmcentrez). Doctors are only allowed to "help" people using a tightly controlled and very specific set of legalized, monopolistic tools that treat symptoms rather than solve the root problem. And if they don't use those tools they can lose their medical license and even get thrown in jail. I've read that the majority of Oncologists wouldn't even treat their own family members with the treatment that they are forced to recommend to their patients. America's healthcare system is like a "house of cards" that could topple at any moment. People aren't taught what their body really needs in the first place, then trillions are spent treating these ailments for a lifetime that shouldn't even exist in the first place. There's no way you're living your best life possible being dependent on this system. That's why it's so important to learn what your body really needs - in the first place. It's all very easy, but our healthcare system makes it seem very hard.

And, this is perhaps the most bizarre, twisted and shameful fact of all. When a commercial airliner crashes anywhere in the world or if even a single American soldier is killed, it always headlines the evening news in America, as it should. Imagine the incredible outrage and urgency there would be to solve the problem if a jumbo jet crashed each and every day in America, killing everyone on board. The President would be giving emergency speeches each day trying to calm everyone down. There would be a 24/7 media coverage on every channel. Airlines would be cancelling flights. Trauma specialists would be meeting with children in schools. America would be gripped in fear and panic. Yet, that's how many people die *each day* in America – a jumbo jet full of American citizens – from *properly prescribed* prescription medicines. And, you hear absolutely nothing about it in the media. Could this be because up to 70% or more of their advertisers are heath care related companies? Then, if that wasn't enough, law makers in Washington have the audacity to try to get bills passed to "save" people from the "dangers" of natural supplements when not a single person has ever died from taking them (http://healthfreedoms.org/2010/03/24/no-deaths-from-vitamins-minerals-amino-acids-or-herbs/). Obviously, the primary goal is to protect industry, not you and your family. This article sums it up nicely: http://www.thenhf.com/article.php?id=486.

Here's another example. Most experts agree that the war on illegal drugs has been a colossal failure. America spends billions of dollars each year trying to stop suppliers of illegal drugs when the goal should be to stop demand by figuring out why people feel the need to take drugs in the first place. The message drilled into our heads is "drugs are bad" or "this is your brain on drugs". Then, you and your family turn on the television and surprisingly, most of the commercials you see are for *drugs*...addictive, man-made legal drugs with lots of side effects that kill more people than illegal drugs! Your children see this, learn that "drugging" yourself is acceptable and the first "option" to consider. Plus, they see mommy and daddy doing it too so it must be o.k. They get hooked on this "solution" even before they're in middle school. Thank goodness only two countries, America and New Zealand, currently allow pharmaceutical advertising on television (http://www.brandweeknrx.com/2007/08/television-drug.html). Note: The primary downside of such prominent pharmaceutical advertising is that it de-incentivizes people to take care of themselves because there is always the illusion that *someone else* will take care of any problems they may develop. There is always a Plan B so it doesn't really matter if they succeed or fail in achieving their health goals. Of course this is great for the healthcare industry but terrible for you.

America, you deserve better. Your family deserves better. You obviously care about your and your family's health. Perhaps you've been too misinformed and don't know exactly what to do and this book will solve that problem for you.

A short while ago I watched a show about Ralph Nader, the legendary consumer advocate. He was asked by the reporter why he had such a passion for getting the truth to consumers about how deceptive companies can be. He said that when he came home from school each day his father's first question to him was always "So, did you learn to *think* today or to believe?" His father wanted him to learn how to think for himself and not simply believe everything he heard or saw. The powers that be don't want you to think, they want you to simply believe. I hope this book gets you to *think*.

I asked a natural health expert what she would do to fix America's healthcare system. She replied "You can't fix it, you simply have to opt-out". I presume she meant the system will never be fixed because there are too many vested interests and too much corruption, complexity and money involved. You simply need to learn how to get and stay healthy easily and inexpensively so you only have to rely on the system for emergency care.

Unfortunately, much of what Western medicine teaches us about how to stay healthy may be dead wrong. Here's an interesting article titled New Study Shows Link Between Statins And Diabetes (http://www.coconutresearchcenter.com/hwnl 9-1.htm) about how cholesterol lowering drugs not only appear to not reduce heart disease – they seem to increase this risk of getting diabetes (which increases the risk of heart disease as well!) and they appear to increase the risk of getting Alzheimer's disease as well! That's because the brain is highly dependent on cholesterol and reducing levels in the blood means there is less for the brain to use. There is no way you can fool your body. No matter what you put in your mouth, your body is going to do the best it can regardless of how many imbalances those products create. The only common sense and humane approach to healthcare for you and your family is to learn what your body needs in the first place by following the checklist at the end of this book. Then give your body what it needs daily for a period of time. If your issues don't improve significantly or resolve themselves after doing this, only *then* should you consider engaging America's healthcare system.

America's healthcare system has been built on the for-profit premise that nutrition has very little to do with disease. Diseases are just something "you get" randomly and since the cause is unknown all you can do is treat the symptoms. Of course this approach, which does not focus on prevention or curing anyone, creates a lifelong stream of highly profitable income for the companies involved. Western trained physicians are apparently taught virtually nothing in medical school about how nutrition affects the human body. Natural medicine, on the other hand, believes that your body is already the most powerful healing force on the planet and is able to heal virtually any disease. All *you* have to do is to simply provide your body the raw materials it needs *in the first place* so balance and harmony can be restored. The belief is that most diseases are caused by your lifestyle choices, so if you simply make better choices and give your body what it needs in the first place, your body will *automatically* correct the issues. You can clearly see how Western medicine and natural medicine compete with each other. You can also see why America's healthcare system would prefer to eliminate the "competition" from natural cures and supplements and there indeed is a bill floating around Washington to try to do just that, called CODEX. This is unfortunate because a country is only comprised of citizens. If those citizens are getting fatter and sicker under the current healthcare paradigm, doing more of the same is only going to make things *worse*. A country is only as strong as its citizens. Sick, fat citizens make for a sick, fat country. So, just be aware that there are invisible forces that exist that do not want you to succeed on your own and they are working against you constantly, much like the undercurrent does when you swim in the ocean. This link pretty much sums up everything you need to know if you are still skeptical that America's healthcare system is not rewarded to prevent disease: http://www4.dr-rath-foundation.org/news-letterlinks/faqs.html#4.

I'm a realist however, and acknowledge that there is certainly a place for pharmaceuticals and medical technology in emergency situations or in those situations where there is absolutely no other option. I just would never recommend them *first* for my own family in those situations where they are clearly not needed and where we can choose a natural option that actually solves the root cause, gives our body what it really needs, is easier and less expensive with no side-effects. Simply treating or suppressing symptoms with pharmaceuticals does nothing to heal the actual root cause.

At this point, is there any doubt in anyone's mind that the American healthcare system is severely broken and completely unsustainable on its current path? Is there any doubt that continuing to follow the advice and methods of this system will not produce the best results in terms of achieving your goals of health, leanness and longevity as easy and inexpensively as possible? Do you really want to pay $15,000 per year for your family's health insurance? Do you want to pay *double* that in just over seven years? I certainly don't and I don't think you do either. Fortunately, these problems are easy and inexpensive to resolve if you just rely on common sense, humanity over profit and honor how your body is designed to work.

The struggle to change America's healthcare system may best be summed up by the following quote:

> *It is difficult to get a man to understand something when his salary depends upon his not understanding it.* - *Upton Sinclair*

This is why it's vital to take your health into your own hands and learn what your body really needs in the first place.

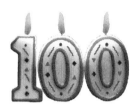

Whose Fault Is It?

America's healthcare system and the health of its citizens are in pretty bad shape. So, what's our natural human inclination? Let's blame someone! It's got to be someone's fault, right?

Many people, including our government, love to blame the pharmaceutical, food, and beverage companies for America's health and obesity problems. I used to think this way as well until something occurred to me. These companies are operating within the boundaries our government sets for them. The government permits the products of these companies to be sold and the majority of the time these companies aren't breaking any laws. Some of their ingredients may also seem suspect at times. But, the government is supposed to monitor ingredients for the safety of American citizens.

The advertising claims of some companies may also be far-fetched, but there's a government agency that monitors that as well. So, if any single group is to blame, it might be our government, right?

You may not know that pharmaceutical advertising is banned in other countries, except for New Zealand. You may also not know that other countries ban foods, ingredients and chemicals that our government allows. Do you ever remember a time when America was the *first* country to ban anything related to food additives or chemicals that we put on or in our body? Other countries ban things all the time that our government allows.

So it *must* be our government's fault, right? Unfortunately, bashing our government or the food, beverage, pharmaceutical or any other industry won't solve our problems.

Here's why:

- No one is forcing you, the American citizen, to use these products.

- There are natural alternatives to pharmaceutical products, as you probably know.

- There are natural and healthy alternatives to man-made, processed foods, fast foods and beverages.

- The burden rests on you, the individual, to know how to read a food label and understand the ingredients used in a product. Just because our government allows it doesn't mean it's good for you. If you can't understand one of the ingredients on a food label, you have the option of not purchasing that product.

- The demand for all products is created by you, the American citizen. The American citizen accounts for 70% of the total spending in this country. If you bought a product, you confirmed your approval for it. If you stopped buying certain products, they would go away because the manufacturer would be forced to adapt by creating products you do want.

- Unless you're being deliberately lied to or deceived or unless someone is forcefully holding you down and stuffing unhealthy products in your mouth and forcing you to swallow them— you and you alone are to blame for the success of almost every industry in America.

It all begins with your choices. Every day you choose what to spend your money on. If you spend your money on something, you're showing your approval for it.

We've all been conditioned to seek the quick-fix. We all want to make our lives easier. But our choices are literally killing us.

If you decide, right now, to change your ways, I promise you it is much easier than you think to achieve your goals. A few Albert Einstein quotes are always helpful to put things in perspective. Here are two of my favorites:

- "We will not solve the problems of today with the level of thinking that created them."

- "All things being equal always choose the simplest solution to a problem."

You know the definition of insanity right? Doing the same thing over and over but expecting a different result! Like Einstein said, to achieve your goals you're going to have to do *something different* in the future than you've done in the past. And, you should concentrate on the *simplest* and most *common sense* solution from this point forward. That's what the remainder of this book is about.

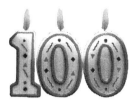

Seven Billion People And Counting

According to the United Nations Population Fund (www. unfpa.org) there are 7 billion people currently on Earth as of November 2011. In 1804 there were only 1 billion people on Earth. So between 1804 and 2011, which is 207 years, Earth's population increased by 6 billion people. That means the population increased by 1 billion people every 34 years on average. However, from this point forward, the United Nations Population Fund estimates that 1 billion people will be added to Earth in just every 12-14 years! That's a rate that's three times faster! In approximately 36 – 42 years Earth's population will increases by another 3 billion people to a total of 10 billion—or about 50% more than it is now!

According to scientists, if you consider natural resource and water supplies, Earth is only capable of supporting about 10 billion people (http://news.yahoo.com/many-people-Earth-support-160802769.html). This article states:

One such scientist, the eminent Harvard University sociobiologist Edward O. Wilson, bases his estimate on calculations of the Earth's available resources. As Wilson pointed out in his book *The Future of Life* (Knopf, 2002):

"The constraints of the biosphere are fixed. Aside from the limited availability of freshwater, there are indeed constraints on the amount of food that Earth can produce, just as Malthus argued more than 200 years ago. Even in the case of maximum efficiency, in which all the grains grown are dedicated to feeding humans (instead of livestock, which is an inefficient way to convert plant energy into food energy), there's still a limit to how far the available quantities can stretch. If everyone agreed to become vegetarian, leaving little or nothing for livestock, the present 1.4 billion hectares of arable land (3.5 billion acres) would support about 10 billion people."

America is estimated to represent about 5% of Earth's population or about 350 million people. In just 12 years that will balloon by another 175 million people to a total of more than 500 million people—about a 50% increase—based on the United Nations' estimates. How can our healthcare system, which is already incredibly inefficient, expensive and unsustainable, support 50% more customers in just another 12 years?

World economies are already deeply in debt and in the midst of a recession, while teetering on the brink of depression. Healthcare costs are skyrocketing at an astronomical rate. People's incomes are stagnant. Companies are pushing more of the costs of healthcare onto the employee. It's like four giant meteors travelling at 29,000 miles per hour that are going to smash into America's healthcare industry in less than 12 years...*unless something changes right now.*

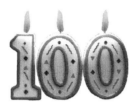

Amazing Facts About Your Amazing Body

Before we get into the details of how your body works and what it needs for simple health, leanness and longevity, I thought it might be interesting to review just how amazing your body really is. Your body is truly a miracle at every level and is certainly worth taking care of. Unfortunately, too many people seem to take their health for granted until they become ill.

There are thousands of facts about the human body on the internet which are certain to leave you curious and in awe. I have listed just some of the ones below that my family and I find fascinating.

- Your body is designed to live in good health to the age of 120-140. Like a modern jetliner gets rebuilt many times over its lifetime, so does your body. Your body is constantly growing "new" organs and cells to replace old ones every second of every day.

- Your body contains about 100 trillion cells which are composed of about 200 different types of cells.

- The length of the blood vessels in your body would total nearly 60,000 miles if they were laid end to end. That's more than two times the distance around Earth at the equator!

- Around 2,000 gallons of blood is pumped through your blood vessels every day (2,000 gallons is about 40 bathtubs filled to the top).

- Your lungs contain around 300 million tiny blood vessels known as capillaries. If these blood vessels were laid end to end, they could stretch over 1,500 miles (that's about halfway across the United States).

- Your lungs inhale about 2 million liters of air each day. If you unfolded your lungs and laid them flat they would cover an area the size of a tennis court.

- Your nose can remember around 50,000 different scents with ease.

- Your heart beats about 130,000 times per day, about 47 million times each year and about 3.7 billion times in a lifetime (a lifetime is 78 years on average).

- Your heart creates so much pressure it can squirt blood over 30 feet.

- Your brain contains about 100 billion neurons.

- Your empty stomach is about the same size as your fist, but it can stretch to about the size of a football.

- Your brain is 60% fat.

- Your blood circulates through your body about three times every minute. In just one day, your blood travels about 12,000 miles. That's four times the distance across the United States.

- Your skeleton weighs between 30%-40% of your total body weight if you are near your ideal weight. So a lean 200 pound man's skeleton would weigh 60 – 80 pounds.

- Pound per pound, your body produces five times more energy than the sun.

- Your brain continues sending electrical wave signals for 37 hours after you die.

- You have fewer bones as an adult than you had as a baby. During infancy there were 350 bones present in your body, but as you grow the bones fuse, and by the time you reached adulthood you have only 206 bones.

- At least 500 species of bacteria, weighing about a total of 3.3 pounds, live inside the human gut.

- Skin is the largest organ of the body. The skin of an adult man can cover an area of approximately 20 sq. ft.

- The acids present in your stomach are strong enough to digest zinc. If your stomach was not capable of continuously producing new stomach lining, these strong acids would digest your stomach.

- A single brain cell has the capacity to store as much information as there is in five encyclopedias.

- About 85% of your immune system is located in your intestines.

- A single block of your bone about the size of a small matchbox has the capacity to support a whopping nine tons (18,000 pounds or about 4 SUV's!).

- Your body can give off enough heat to boil a gallon of water within half an hour.

- Of all the oxygen you breathe, 20% goes to your brain.

- In one day you shed around 10 billion skin flakes.

- Every square inch of your body has about 19 million skin cells.

- Every hour your body replaces 1 billion cells.

- Your small intestine is about two inches around and 20 feet long.

- Your body makes one to three pints of saliva every 24 hours. In a lifetime that can fill two large swimming pools.

- If you are cremated when you die, about 96% of your ashes would be minerals.

- Your body has about 37,000 miles of capillaries.

- Capillaries are so small it takes about 10 of them to equal the thickness of a single human hair. However, your aorta, which is the largest artery in your body, is about the diameter of a garden hose.

- Your body needs about 88 pounds of oxygen each day.

- Your eye can detect 500 shades of gray, up to 1 million surface colors and can take in more information than the largest telescope known to man.

- Although bones are hard on the outside, they are generally soft and light on the inside. They are about 75% water.

- Your body can live for about 40 days without food, about seven days without water and about six to eight minutes without oxygen.

- The acidity of your stomach is about 100,000 times greater than the acidity of your bloodstream.

- Each cell in your body contains an estimated six to eight feet of DNA. If the DNA in your body was laid end to end it would stretch across our entire solar system. (The distance is calculated by multiplying 100 trillion cells in your body times about seven feet of DNA in each cell. That's 700 trillion feet of DNA in your body, divided by the number of feet in a mile which is 5,280. So the answer is over 132 million miles. The sun is about 93 million miles away so the length of the DNA in your body would stretch from Earth to 40 million miles past the sun!)

- If the information in your DNA was written down, it would fill 1,000 encyclopedias.

- Your brain is capable of having more ideas than the number of atoms in the known universe.

- About 50 million cells in your body will have died and been replaced by the time you read this sentence.

- Your hearing is so sensitive it can distinguish between hundreds of thousands of sounds.

- When you touch something you send messages to your brain at 124 miles per hour.

- Nerve impulses are sent through our body at around 248 miles per hour.

- Your body contains over 600 muscles.

- The average lifespan of a single taste bud is 10 days.

- Your body contains enough carbon to manufacture 900 pencils.

- Without your big toes you would simply fall over.

- If you could save all the times you blink in a lifetime and use them all at once you would see blackness for 1.2 years.

- In one hour your heart produces the energy equivalent to raise a one ton weight (2,000 pounds) three feet off the ground. The strongest human in history can only lift around 800 pounds.

- You would have to walk 50 miles to equal the amount of exercise your eyes get in a single day.

- Your body is able to heal itself from virtually anything unless you keep injuring it.

I hope you agree that your body is an absolutely miraculous gift that's worth taking care of.

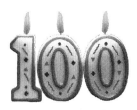

What Constitutes Health? Fitness? Aging? Wellness? Longevity?

Since we are striving for these things, let's first learn what they mean.

Health:
The absence of physical and mental disease. This includes all physical diseases as well as all mental and emotional diseases, such as depression, addictions, compulsions, etc.

Fitness:
The capacity to perform physical activities without getting tired.

(How fit you are is not a reliable indicator of how healthy you are or how long you will live, unfortunately.)

Aging:
Aging is when your body wears out faster than it re-builds itself.

Wellness:
The overall state of being in good mental, physical, and emotional health.

Longevity:
Your lifespan from the moment of your birth (point A) to the moment your heart stops beating (point B). When I use the word longevity in this book, I am referring to reaching at least 100 years of age.

Remember, though, that Healthy Lifespan refers to the number of years you live *without* a debilitating condition. A goal of this book is to make sure your Healthy Lifespan exceeds 100 years of age as well. There's no use living to 100 years of age if the last 20 years of your life are spent in and out of hospitals.

Leanness:
The condition of having visible muscle tone and appropriate body fat for your age. People who are lean have better and more visible muscle tone than people who are simply "skinny." You can be skinny and "flabby" at the same time. Leanness is measured using your body fat percentage, as is described in a coming chapter. Lean does not mean you have to be "ripped" or "defined" like a body builder.

(Unfortunately, your level of leanness is not a reliable indicator of your health or potential lifespan.)

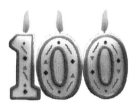

Distractions: The Latest Health Studies

I wish to address this point before we move forward—all those new health studies and breakthroughs we constantly hear about. Just about every week in America there's a new study discussed on the media about the latest health revelation. Be aware that these studies are, for the most part, distractions. They create a knee-jerk reaction in people. "Hey, that sounds good, that must be what I'm missing," they think. Often the results of that study become the new health fad and further distract people from the real answers. With so much focus on *new, new, new* it's easy to lose focus of the basics, the fundamentals and the entire foundation that must be put in place first so you can easily achieve your goals. As you will learn in an upcoming chapter, it's silly to run out and buy products that these studies recommend when up to 95% of us aren't even providing our body with the absolute basic spectrum of raw materials it needs every day to do its job properly.

To determine whether the newest study's advice is valid or

not, ask yourself one simple question:

- Is there any healthy, long-lived group of people on Earth who don't follow this advice yet are still healthier than Americans? (If the answer is "yes" don't believe the study.)

Here are some examples we've heard about in the past:

- <u>Don't eat coconut oil.</u> Years ago in America it was thought that coconut oil and palm oil were evil for the body because they are among the most saturated of fats and a flawed study suggested saturated fats cause heart disease. Yet all over the world, especially in tropical climates, people have eaten large amounts of coconut oil for thousands of years yet are much healthier with far less heart disease than Americans. We should have never believed this from the beginning because it didn't pass our simple question test.

- <u>Don't eat butter.</u> Pretty much the same flawed saturated fat story as coconut oil, but the myth continues on popular medical news shows and in the media even to this day. Are the countries of the world that consume a lot of butter dying faster than Americans? No. The French are one of the largest consumers of butter and they have less heart disease than Americans. Again, asking this simple question would have eliminated years of confusion and health problems.

- <u>Don't eat eggs.</u> Eggs contain cholesterol and it was thought that eating foods high in cholesterol raised cholesterol levels in your body and caused plaque in your arteries. Most experts to-day don't believe this as they know about 80% of the cholesterol your body needs is made by your liver, but the myth still continues. A whole industry of "egg substitutes" has sprung up. Are longer living cultures around the world avoiding eggs? No.

- <u>Stay out of the sun.</u> Americans have one of the highest skin cancer rates in the world yet we spend among the least time in the sun. So, do cultures that spend a lot time in the sun die from skin cancer more than Americans? No. Out of 192 countries, America ranks 29th high-est in skin cancer. That means the citizens of 163 countries get *less* skin cancer than Ameri-cans and many of them spend much more time in the sun than Americans do.

My point is this—the next time you hear about the latest, greatest health breakthrough in the media, ask yourself the simple question above. Your health and life may de-pend on it.

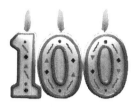

They Often
Perpetuate Myths

Perhaps nothing frustrates me more than watching a TV personality—someone who has a show that attracts millions of viewers—spout out recycled, tired or incorrect health advice. It happens all the time on popular morning television shows. It happens all the time on informational doctor shows. The problem is—it happens all the time!

For example, if you ever hear a health expert on TV say that saturated fat causes heart disease please, please, please tell them to read a book by Bruce Fife, N.D. called *Saturated Fat May Save Your Life*. Saturated fats don't cause heart disease. It's a myth. Yet it's still spouted all the time on TV. The public blindly accepts this information as fact because of who's dishing it out and it harms real people.

Many mistakes are spouted by people on TV and radio shows about cholesterol, saturated fat, heart disease, cancer causes or the need (or lack of need) for certain nutrients. These myths trickle down through our society and the myths remain alive and can negatively affect the view-ers' health. It confuses society and helps perpetuate our health and obesity problems.

Please be wary of any information you hear on these shows and do your own research. Many times these people on TV are hired due to their 'likability factor,' not because they know what they are talking about.

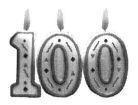

What Really Determines The Way You Look, Feel And Perform

Health experts state that about 85% of the way you look, feel, perform and how long you live is determined by what you choose to put in your mouth. This includes foods, beverages, medicines, herbs, spices and whatever else you can eat. You really are what you eat and there's no getting around it. It's worth repeating—85% of the way you look (weight, fat, hair, nails, skin, muscle tone, complexion, etc.), how you feel (your health, energy levels, mental sharpness, ability to deal with stress, emotional stability, etc.) and how long you live is determined by what you choose to put in your mouth. The important word here is *choose*. Nothing hops in your mouth automatically or against your will. If it's in your mouth you put it there. If you swallow it, that was your choice too.

That means the remaining 15% of how you look, feel,

perform and how long you live is determined by every-thing *other* than what you choose to put in your mouth. This includes your genetics, general activity level, exer-cise level, how well you sleep, etc.

The point is, if you can control what you choose to put in your mouth you've already achieved 85% of your health, weight and longevity goals! So, if the potential human lifespan is 120 years, 85% of that is 102 years—achieved simply by controlling what you choose to put in your mouth.

It is astonishing to think of all the industries, products and services that exist in America today (including our massive healthcare system) that result primarily from one thing—people not being able to control what they put in their mouth!

It all starts with what you choose to put in your mouth. That's the first step—the first domino. Depending on what you put in your mouth determines the direction that first domino falls. Which direction it falls deter-mines the path your health, weight and longevity will take.

This is very important to remember as we move for-ward. Your primary goal is to control what you put in your mouth. Period. Although this may be difficult for you to do now, when you learn how your body actually works you will find it very easy. Amazingly easy!

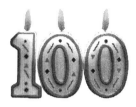

How Much Should You Weigh?

Another bit of housekeeping I want to get out of the way is how much you should weigh. There are many tables like the one below that can be found on the internet that show how much you should weigh based on your height and frame size. As the table correctly states, you need to know your frame size first. To calculate your frame size, do the following:

- Measure the size of your wrist using your hand. If you are left-handed, measure your right wrist. If you are right-handed, measure your left wrist.

- Wrap your free hand around your wrist and try to touch your middle finger to your thumb.

Small Frame: If your middle finger and thumb overlap, you have a small frame.

Medium Frame: If your middle finger and thumb touch, you have a medium frame.

Large Frame: If your middle finger and thumb do not touch, you have a large frame.

WOMEN				MEN			
Height	**Frame Size**			**Height**	**Frame Size**		
Ft. In.	**Small**	**Med.**	**Large**	**Ft. In.**	**Small**	**Med.**	**Large**
4'10"	102-111	109-121	118-131	5'2"	128-134	131-141	138-150
4'11"	103-113	111-123	120-134	5'3"	130-136	133-143	140-153
5'0"	104-115	113-126	122-137	5'4"	132-138	135-145	142-156
5'1"	106-118	115-129	125-140	5'5"	134-140	137-148	144-160
5'2"	108-121	118-132	128-143	5'6"	136-142	139-151	146-164
5'3"	111-124	121-135	131-147	5'7"	138-145	142-154	149-168
5'4"	114-127	124-138	134-151	5'8"	140-148	145-157	152-172
5'5"	117-130	127-141	137-155	5'9"	142-151	156-160	155-176
5'6"	120-133	130-144	140-159	5'10"	144-154	151-163	158-180
5'7"	123-136	133-144	143-163	5'11"	146-157	154-166	161-184
5'8"	126-139	136-150	146-167	6'0"	149-160	157-170	164-188
5'9"	129-142	139-153	149-170	6'1"	152-164	160-174	168-192
5'10"	132-145	142-156	152-173	6'2"	155-168	165-178	172-197
5'11"	135-148	145-159	155-176	6'3"	158-172	167-182	176-202
6'0"	138-151	148-162	158-176	6'4"	162-176	171-187	181-207

I recommend that you never use the popular BMI (Body Mass Index) to determine whether you are overweight or not. That's because the BMI's fatal flaw is that it does not discriminate between where the weight comes from—muscle, fat, bone density or water. Because of this flaw very muscular people, including bodybuilders, can be considered obese using the BMI. Yet according to other more relevant measures, these people are highly fit and trim with very little body fat. Likewise, people who are within their ideal BMI range can have a dangerously high percentage of body fat and actually be very "flabby."

A much better measurement is to use your body fat percentage. You measure your body fat percentage using a special scale you can buy at most sporting goods stores or using a device called a caliper.

For example, AccuFitness is the maker of the popular <u>Accu-Measure Body Fat Caliper</u> which is a one site skin fold body fat measurement method. When you buy the product, AccuFitness includes body fat percentage charts like the ones below for men and women. They are based on research by Jackson & Pollock, and have become the industry standard. Charts like the ones below can be found on various websites. You can buy the AccuFitness calipers at many stores or on their website at <u>www.accufitness.com</u>.

Notice that weight does not matter in these charts. If a man weighs 200 pounds and is 5'5" tall, he would be considered obese using the BMI. Yet if that same man is 54 years old and has only 8.8% body fat, he would be considered extremely lean using the body fat percentage calculation. The point is, use body fat percentage and the below tables to accurately determine whether you are lean, average or above average in terms of body fat. Do not use BMI or weight alone.

BODY FAT % MEASUREMENT CHART FOR MEN
Accu-Measure™ Reading in Millimeters

AGE	2-3	4-5	6-7	8-9	10-11	12-13	14-15	16-17	18-19	20-21	22-23	24-25	26-27	28-29	30-31	32-33	34-36
18-20	2.0	3.9	6.2	8.5	10.5	12.5	14.3	16.0	17.5	18.9	20.2	21.3	22.3	23.1	23.8	24.3	24.9
21-25	2.5	4.9	7.3	9.5	11.6	13.6	15.4	17.0	18.6	20.0	21.2	22.3	23.3	24.2	24.9	25.4	25.8
26-30	3.5	6.0	8.4	10.6	12.7	14.6	16.4	18.1	19.6	21.0	22.3	23.4	24.4	25.2	25.9	26.5	26.9
31-35	4.5	7.1	9.4	11.7	13.7	15.7	17.5	19.2	20.7	22.1	23.4	24.5	25.5	26.3	27.0	27.5	28.0
36-40	5.6	8.1	10.5	12.7	14.8	16.8	18.6	20.2	21.8	23.2	24.4	25.6	26.5	27.4	28.1	28.6	29.0
41-45	6.7	9.2	11.5	13.8	15.9	17.8	19.6	21.3	22.8	24.7	25.5	26.6	27.6	28.4	29.1	29.7	30.1
46-50	7.7	10.2	12.6	14.8	16.9	18.9	20.7	22.4	23.9	25.3	26.6	27.7	28.7	29.5	30.2	30.7	31.2
51-55	8.8	11.3	13.7	15.9	18.0	20.0	21.8	23.4	25.0	26.4	27.6	28.7	29.7	30.6	31.2	31.8	32.2
56 & UP	9.9	12.4	14.7	17.0	19.1	21.0	22.8	24.5	26.0	27.4	28.7	29.8	30.8	31.6	32.3	32.9	33.3
	LEAN				IDEAL				AVERAGE				ABOVE AVERAGE				

BODY FAT % MEASUREMENT CHART FOR WOMEN
Accu-Measure® Reading in Millimeters

AGE	2-3	4-5	6-7	8-9	10-11	12-13	14-15	16-17	18-19	20-21	22-23	24-25	26-27	28-29	30-31	32-33	34-36
18-20	11.3	13.5	15.7	17.7	19.7	21.5	23.2	24.8	26.3	27.7	29.0	30.2	31.3	32.3	33.1	33.9	34.6
21-25	11.9	14.2	16.3	18.4	20.3	22.1	23.8	25.5	27.0	28.4	29.6	30.8	31.9	32.9	33.8	34.5	35.2
26-30	12.5	14.8	16.9	19.0	20.9	22.7	24.5	26.1	27.6	29.0	30.3	31.5	32.5	33.5	34.4	35.2	35.8
31-35	13.2	15.4	17.6	19.6	21.5	23.4	25.1	26.7	28.2	29.6	30.9	32.1	33.2	34.1	35.0	35.8	36.4
36-40	13.8	16.0	18.2	20.2	22.2	24.0	25.7	27.3	28.8	30.2	31.5	32.7	33.8	34.8	35.6	36.4	37.0
41-45	14.4	16.7	18.8	20.8	22.8	24.6	26.3	27.9	29.4	30.8	32.1	33.3	34.4	35.4	36.3	37.0	37.7
46-50	15.0	17.3	19.4	21.5	23.4	25.2	26.9	28.6	30.1	31.5	32.8	34.0	35.0	36.0	36.9	37.6	38.3
51-55	15.6	17.9	20.0	22.1	24.0	25.9	27.6	29.2	30.7	32.1	33.4	34.6	35.6	36.6	37.5	38.3	38.9
56 & UP	16.3	18.5	20.7	22.7	24.6	26.5	28.2	29.8	31.3	32.7	34.0	35.2	36.3	37.2	38.1	38.9	39.5
	LEAN				IDEAL				AVERAGE				ABOVE AVERAGE				

Note that the vertical scale on the left side of the chart is age. The scale across the bottom of the chart measures body fat percentage.

Also note that as you age you are allowed to have a higher body fat percentage and still remain in a particular category. For example, a woman between the ages of 21-25 with a body fat percentage of 26.5 would be "average" on the leanness scale. Yet when that same woman is age 56 or older and at 26.5% body fat, that puts her right at the edge of the lean category. Your measure of leanness is dynamic and based on a combination of your age and body fat percentage.

Remember, your body *needs* a certain percentage of body fat to be optimally healthy and too little body fat can be just as dangerous as too much body fat.

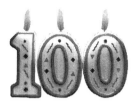

The Number Of Calories You Need

Eating should be natural, enjoyable and stress free. You shouldn't have to count anything as that takes all the fun out of it. Nor should you have to punish yourself or feel guilty for your inability to eat perfectly all the time.

There are two ways your body burns calories - Basal Metabolic Rate and "Everything Else".

<u>Basal Metabolic Rate (BMR)</u>: If you lie on the couch watching TV or sleeping for 24 hours straight your body is still burning calories to keep you alive. Even though you have no movement or activity your body generally burns around 11 calories per pound of body weight through the beating of your heart, unconscious activity of your brain, breathing, etc. So, if you weigh 200 pounds you would burn around 2,200 calories a day (200 lbs. x 11 calories per pound). Your BMR accounts for about 75% of the total calories you burn each day.

You will often hear that building more muscle mass increases your BMR. If you have more muscle, you will burn more calories doing nothing (your BMR will be higher) than you will if you have less muscle. But remember, when you exercise you will often get hungrier than if you do not exercise because your body wants to replace the lost fuel it just burned. Building muscle requires effort. Effort requires fuel. And that fuel comes from eating more calories. Some argue that the net result of exercise (in terms of weight loss) is a net neutral activity. That is, the extra calories you burn while exercising are often eaten later because you're hungrier *from* exercising. Other people eat less after they exercise. You will have to listen to your body to learn how it responds.

Everything Else: If your BMR accounts for approximately 75% of the total calories you burn each day (about 11 calories per pound), then everything else accounts for approximately 25% of the total calories you burn or about an additional three calories per pound. Everything else means whatever else you normally do when you're not lying on the couch watching TV; things like your general activity level, exercise level, stress level, etc.

How Many Calories Do You Need in Total?

The total calories that will permit you to maintain your weight are your BMR of 11 calories per pound plus your 'Everything Else' category of 3 calories per pound for a grand total of 14 calories per pound. Keep in mind this is an approximate number and can deviate up or down a few calories if you are at either extreme end of the activity spectrum. So, if you weigh 200 pounds and you wish to maintain your weight, you can consume 2,880 calories per day (200 pounds times 14 calories per pound).

You've probably heard before that it takes a deficit of 3,500 calories to lose one pound of weight (not fat). Therefore, if you reduce your total weekly caloric intake by 3,500 calories (500 calories a day for 7 days, for example) you will lose one pound of weight. The pound of weight you lose will consist of approximately 80% muscle and water and 20% fat. To lose weight, first start by identifying your target weight. For example, if you currently weigh 200 pounds and your goal is to weigh 160 pounds in the future, you should begin consuming the number of calories *now* as though you already weigh 160 pounds and are simply trying to maintain that weight. So rather than taking in 2,800 calories per day (200 lbs. x 14 calories per pound) you would take in 2,240 calories per day (160 lbs. x 14 calories per pound) and that would allow you to gradually lose weight without feeling deprived until you reached your goal of 160 lbs. Once you reached your goal of 160 pounds, simply continue to consume 14 calories per pound to maintain that weight.

What if You Only Want to Lose Fat?

I recall hearing a famous plastic surgeon talking about liposuction on a radio show a few years ago. He indicated that if he removes 10 pounds of fat through liposuction, that really is all fat with just a tiny bit of blood. He compared that to losing 10 pounds of weight. He said about eight pounds or 80% of that would be muscle and water and only two pounds (20%) would be fat. The point is you can't lose just fat on your own. Nothing spot reduces fat other than a medical procedure. In the above example, to lose 10 pounds of fat, you'd have to lose 50 pounds of total weight. That's because 50 pounds times 20% equals 10 pounds of fat. Forty pounds of your weight loss would come from muscle and water loss.

Keep this in mind that any weight you lose will be comprised of about 20% fat and 80% muscle and water. This is discouraging for sure, but something worth keeping in mind as you continue.

No Need To Count Macronutrients

Fat, protein, and carbohydrates are the only source of calories for humans. They are called macronutrients and are usually measured in grams. Grams of weight are converted to their caloric equivalent as follows:

- One gram of fat contains nine calories.

- One gram of protein or carbohydrate contains approximately four calories.

At first glance, if your goal is to lose weight, you would naturally conclude that you should eat less fat because fat contains twice the calories per gram as protein or carbohydrates, right? But, researchers know that's no longer true. The old formula of total calories in minus total calories out isn't really accurate. It's what your body decides to do with those calories—store them or shed them—that matters. So what might cause your body to store excess calories when another person's body sheds those excess calories? You will learn the answer in a coming chapter.

Quite a few books have been published on the optimal ratio of protein, fats and carbohydrates you should consume each day. I never placed much value on these ratios as, again, they seem to be of little value in my research. I have a *Navy Seal Workout* book on my bookshelf I purchased a number of years ago. You would think Navy Seals would consume a lot of protein, right? Their diet, at least the way I calculated it, is only about 12%-20% protein. And what group of us normal working humans is more physically or mentally stressed than Navy Seals? None!

Dr. Joel Fuhrman, author of *Eat To Live*, indicates most people actively seek out protein sources because of all the hype you hear in the media. He says the only way you won't get enough protein in your diet, even if you are a vegetarian, is if you're actually *starving to death*. He indicates plants provide more protein than steak, on an adjusted basis. I would highly recommend reading his book as it covers in detail some of the principles of eating covered in this book.

If you're interested in having a target to aim for, I can only tell you what seems to work for my family. I would guess we eat around:

- 15%-20% protein (mostly from vegetables, fruits, legumes, nuts, seeds, raw dairy, whole grains and some meats)

- 30% or more healthy fats (mostly from nuts, seeds, butter, coconut oil, olive oil, raw dairy)

- Roughly 50% carbohydrates (mostly from fruits, vegetables, legumes, rice, whole grains)

I have read of cultures that eat as much as 70% fat, few if any carbohydrates and 30% protein and they are perfectly healthy. You can read more about these cultures on Dr. Weston Price's website or through his landmark book *Nutrition & Physical Degeneration* in the Resources section.

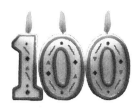

Review Of What You've Learned So Far

Before we dive into the details that you've been waiting for, let's review the preliminary groundwork you've learned so far so it's fresh in your mind. This preliminary information will serve as the foundation for the remaining information in this book.

So far you've learned:

- The American healthcare system is designed to treat disease, not prevent it

- Personal responsibility is absolutely imperative in your quest to achieve your goals

- Your lifespan will average 78 years if you live in America

- You will most certainly die from one of the top 15 causes of death—most of which are completely avoidable

- What the longest lived people in the world have in common

- How much you should weigh based on your frame size and height

- What your body fat percentage should be and how to measure it

- How many calories you need to maintain or lose weight

- That approximately 85% of the way you look and feel is determined by what you choose to eat and drink

- That about 75% of the total calories you burn each day are from your Basal Metabolic Rate and the remaining 25% of the calories you burn are due to your general activity/exercise level

- Counting calories and grams of protein, fat or carbohydrates is not necessary if you give your body the raw materials it needs first

- To focus on the basics of what has kept humans alive for thousands of years and to essentially ignore the latest, greatest health studies

- Getting lean or exercising are not good indicators of disease avoidance or increased longevity

- You can't spot reduce fat

- Facts about how truly amazing your body really is

- That you get fat, sick, age and die due to imbalances in your body and these imbalances are virtually all due to your choices

Coming up next you'll learn how you can easily control what you put in your mouth and how to fix your metabolism easily and inexpensively.

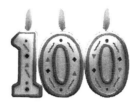

Why You Get Hungry

Finally we get to the eating part! Ok, you're hungry—what's your body asking for? First consider this somewhat strange thought—you are not hungry. Your body—that machine you live in that keeps you alive—is hungry. When you travel as a passenger in a car and the car needs fuel, you don't need fuel. The machine you're riding in needs fuel—same concept with hunger. Let's assume you are riding in a machine in this lifetime called your body.

So what is your body asking for when it's hungry? Let's think about it. Your body can *only* be asking for one or more of the following when you feel hungry:

- Water (your body can sometimes confuse hunger with thirst)

- Calories (from the macronutrients—protein, fat, and carbohydrates)

- Micronutrients (vitamins, minerals, amino acids, essential fatty acids)

That's it! Let's take a closer look at what your body might be asking for when you feel hungry:

- <u>Water</u>. Maybe you're just thirsty. Sometimes you think you're hungry when you're simply thirsty. A weight loss expert and therapist I know always drinks a glass of water first every time he feels hungry, then he waits 15 minutes. If he still feels hungry after 15 minutes he eats because he knows it was true hunger, not just thirst masking itself as hunger.

- <u>Calories</u>. You simply may not be eating enough macronutrient calories in the form of protein, carbohydrates or fat to fuel your body's burn rate of about 14 calories per pound. If you need 2,800 calories per day based on your weight and you've only eaten 1,000 calories so far that day, your body may signal hunger because it simply needs more calories to support cellular functions.

- <u>Micronutrients</u>. Macronutrients contain things called micronutrients. These are vitamins, minerals, amino acids, and essential fatty acids. Your body might be asking for any or all of the micronutrients. If you happen to eat macronutrients that don't contain any micronutrients that's referred to as "empty calories" because you are consuming only calories and nothing else of value. This is a big problem in America since experts estimate that 90% of the food Americans eat is processed.

That's all your body could be asking for when you feel hunger. So, of those possible choices, which one(s) might actually be <u>causing</u> your body's hunger if you're a typical American? Let's think about it. If you're like most Americans:

- <u>Are you dehydrated and suffering from a lack of water?</u> Possibly, but remember you get hydrated from the water in foods and beverages too, not just by drinking eight cups of water each day. If you don't feel thirsty you are probably not dehydrated. Some would disagree but remember, you must listen to your body. Many countries around the world live longer than Americans and only drink when they are thirsty. Research is also suggesting that too much water is actually adding to our health problems. You will learn why in an upcoming chapter.

- <u>Are you suffering from a lack of calories in the form of fat, carbohydrates, or protein?</u> Probably not as most Americans already eat far too many calories.

- <u>Are you suffering from a lack of micronutrients (vitamins, minerals, amino acids, essential fatty acids)?</u> YES! Why does this matter? You will learn why in a coming chapter.

Remember, your body only signals hunger for two primary reasons:

- It needs calories from macronutrients
- It needs micronutrients

This is *vitally* important to keep in mind as we continue.

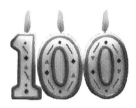

Why People Eat
Too Many Calories
Yet Are Still Hungry

What really determines how much you eat or when you stop eating? How can some people stuff themselves and then just moments later be hungry or crave something else? Our health problems and expanding waistlines prove that the number of calories we consume or over-consume do not seem to stop our urge to eat. Most people are always hungry and they don't know why. They've definitely eaten plenty of calories—that's for sure. Unfortunately, hunger doesn't just stop once you've eaten the right amount of calories your body needs. If it did, none of us would be overweight.

Your stomach is about the size of your clenched fist. If you look at your fist right now you'll see that it may not look particularly large in comparison to the volume of food you may eat. That's because your stomach is able to stretch to about the size of a football!

There are a number of theories about how the signals to stop eating get triggered. Some of the more popular ones are:

Eating high volume foods. One theory about what signals you to stop eating involves the volume of food you've eaten. The belief is that the volume of the food you've eaten stretches the stomach and that stretching signals you to stop eating. So eating a large salad should make you feel fuller quicker than eating a four ounce piece of steak, which is about the size of a deck of playing cards. If you've ever eaten a large salad and still felt hungry or craved something only moments later you know this volume theory is not always true.

Fiber falls into this category of increasing volume and thereby helps you to feel full faster. If the goal was only to increase volume then you would never have to eat anything—you could simply drink a large volume of water when you are hungry and that alone would stop your hunger. If you've ever tried this you know that it does not work that way. Many people I know have tried drinking a large amount of water before a meal and they still seem to eat as much. Others drink large amounts of a beverage with a meal. That's bad because it dilutes your stomach acid, can result in undigested food passing into your intestines and can wash away precious nutrients.

Eating physically heavy foods. Another theory about why we stop eating is the belief that it's the physical weight of the food you've eaten that signals you to stop eating. Eating heavy, dense foods should make you feel fuller faster. Of course heavy foods tend to be calorie dense foods as well. But, as long as the foods you're eating are whole, natural foods and not processed, this may work to some degree.

<u>Eating slowly</u>. You've been told to eat slowly because it takes about 20 minutes for your brain and stomach to communicate that you're full. If you've ever tried to eat slowly, you may find it works. If you consume a high calorie meal in just a few minutes, the thought is that you're eating many more calories than you otherwise might have had you eaten more slowly. When I was a teenager, I remember seeing a headline in a grocery store tabloid that trumpeted a "miracle" new way to lose weight. The miracle? Eat using chopsticks so you eat more slowly.

<u>Chewing your food longer</u>. Another theory is that the simple act of chewing is what triggers signals to stop eating. Chew your food 20 times until it turns to mush and you lose weight, right? Then how do you explain becoming hungry after chewing a piece of gum all afternoon?

<u>Eating a large variety of foods</u>. Another theory involves the variety of foods you eat at a given meal. The thinking is the more flavors and aromas you experience during a meal, the faster you will be satisfied. So if you are eating from a smorgasbord or buffet, you should eat less and become fuller faster. If you've ever been on a cruise ship, you know this theory doesn't always work as many people eat themselves silly and end up gaining quite a bit of weight during the cruise.

<u>Eating strong smelling foods</u>. How about the theory that eating foods that have strong smells and that are very aromatic will make you stop eating sooner? Taste is said to be about 85% smell so this makes some sense, right? I'm sure you or your children have taken a medicine or eaten something that tastes terrible, but if you hold your nose while swallowing you can barely taste it. If this theory was true, then all the cultures that eat aromatic foods or spices would all be very slender. They're not.

Eating more fat. Another theory involves the amount of fat you consume. Fat is naturally satiating and contains about double the calories per gram as carbohydrates or protein. Therefore, by adding fat to your meal, you will turn off hunger signals faster, right? This makes some sense but many people can eat an entire bag of potato chips consisting of a thousand calories from fat and still remain hungry afterwards. According to Dr. Michael Green, a research psychologist at Aston University, our brains are made up of 60% fat. To function optimally our brains need to maintain this level of fat. A lower amount of fat, in fact, can lead to neurological disorders. So, eating more fat seems to make sense as long as it's the right kind of fat. The key is being able to stop yourself before you consume too many calories.

The point I'm trying to make is that no one seems to know for sure what turns off hunger signals and what ultimately makes you stop eating. They all seem to work to some degree. But all of the above tips, theories, and beliefs have been around for years and they don't seem to be making us any thinner or healthier. That means there must be *something else* that matters in shutting down or regulating your hunger. I'll explain what pioneering health experts believe it is in the next chapter.

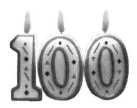

The Magic Of
The 100 Buckets

I'd like you to try to put your conscious thoughts and beliefs aside for a moment. Forget about taste, emotions or
stress. Just pretend you are a cell in your body and your
only goal is to survive by obtaining what you need, selfish
as that may sound.

What are the absolute minimum things you need as a cell
in order to survive?

- Oxygen

- Water

- Freedom from toxins

- Calories (macronutrients)

- Micronutrients (vitamins, minerals, amino acids, essential fatty acids)

Let's say you decide to put something in your mouth—food or beverage—it doesn't matter. As that food or beverage passes into your stomach and small intestine, what's really happening down there? What might your cells and body be thinking? For lack of a better description, let's assume your body begins *scanning* what you just swallowed to see if there is anything worthwhile it can use. What you swallowed leaves your stomach and enters your small intestine where nutrients are absorbed. Imagine there are approximately 100 tiny buckets lined up in your small intestine. There is one bucket for each of the 100 vitamins, minerals, amino acids and essential fatty acids your body needs. *Wait. 100 what?*

That's right, according to top natural health experts, your body needs approximately 100 essential and trace nutrients every day in order to fully switch on your DNA within each cell so your body performs at optimal functioning. These 100 nutrients are the micronutrient raw materials your DNA, cells, metabolism, immune system and body need to fully do their job for you and to make everything operate properly just as it is supposed to.

The term 'essential' refers to those nutrients your body needs for optimal health and functioning but can't make (or can't make in sufficient quantities). The only way you can get them is from your diet. The term 'trace nutrient' refers to those nutrients that are important to healthy functioning and required in very small amounts called micrograms. Everything you put in your mouth (except water) will obviously contain calories from macronutrients. But, depending on the quality and source of those macronutrients, they may contain few if any micronutrients. The term 'empty calories' refers to the eating of macronutrients that contain very few or no micronutrients. In other words, if the majority of what you eat contains only calories with few micronutrients—you are eating empty calories and are most likely gaining weight and are always hungry.

Experts say that 90% of what Americans eat is processed. Processing removes vital nutrients. Eating this way (lots of calories, few micronutrients) will pack on the pounds quickly and lay the foundation for many diseases and imbalances.

The approximately 100 essential and trace nutrients you need every day are:

- 16 Vitamins (15 vitamins plus bioflavonoids)

- 12 Amino Acids

- 3 Essential Fatty Acids (EFA) (if you get two of them your body can make the third)

- 70+ Minerals (Some experts believe we only need 60 minerals while others suggest 70 or 75 or 84. The number of minerals you can obtain is somewhat dependent on the form of the minerals you consume. Throughout this book I will use the minimum of 70 as that is approximately the average within the range. I have never read any research that suggests fewer minerals is better, so in my family we aim for at least 70 when possible.)

Although this sounds like a lot of nutrients each day, in reality, it is not that far off from current recommendations. A typical food label contains recommendations for 27 vitamins and minerals which are comprised of 13 vitamins, six macro minerals and eight essential trace minerals. Then, add in the eight amino acids that are considered essential and the three essential fatty acids and that totals 38 nutrients. The only nutrients that are missing from current recommendations are the full spectrum of 56+ *additional* trace minerals and four additional amino acids. The below table summarizes this comparison:

	Approximate Current Recommendations	Natural Health Expert Recommendations
Vitamins	13	16
Major & Trace Minerals	14	14
Additional Trace Minerals	0	56+
Amino Acids	8	12
EFAs	3	3
Total Nutrients	38	101

I will discuss this in more detail in a later chapter so, for now, let's get back to what's happening in your body after you've eaten something:

> Imagine all the <u>calories</u> from the <u>macronutrients</u> you've just eaten magically pass through the 100 buckets in your small intestine. Your body takes the calories and macronutrients it needs, burns some as energy and if you've eaten too many, stores the rest for later (often as fat).
>
> Next, your body scans the food for <u>micronutrients (vitamins, minerals, amino acids, essential fatty acids)</u>. Every time it finds a nutrient it needs it puts that nutrient into the appropriate nutrient bucket.

After all the calories, macronutrients and micronutrients have been sorted out, here's what your body might say:

Hmmm...

   • <u>*My calorie bucket is full*</u>, *even overflowing. My master has eaten more calories from fats, proteins, and carbohydrates than I need. Let's store some in case we run out of food.*

- *Only 14 of my <u>micronutrient</u> buckets are totally full.*

- *22 of my <u>micronutrient</u> buckets are less than half full.*

- *Over 65 of my <u>micronutrient</u> buckets are still completely empty.*

Ok, I have plenty of calories, fats, carbohydrates, and protein. But, I don't have nearly enough micronutrients, and I need them to keep my master healthy, safe, and happy.

Being that the innate evolutionary wisdom of your body is much smarter than your conscious thoughts, what does your body conclude? It concludes *'I need these vital micronutrients for every single function in my master, to fully switch on my DNA and to successfully do all the jobs I need to do, but I am missing a lot of them. So,*

- *I can either shut a few things down*

- *I can operate at a reduced energy level overall*

- *I can borrow some nutrients from my bones or other organs*

- *Or, I can give my master the signal to stay hungry so he will keep eating and hopefully provide me with these nutrients I need.'*

So your body, with its amazing evolutionary and survival wisdom does a little of each:

- It shuts a few things down

- It operates at a reduced energy level overall

- It borrows some of the nutrients it needs from bones or other organs—thereby creating deficiencies and imbalances in those areas

- It keeps you hungry hoping you'll eat something that contains the nutrients it needs

What has your body just done? It's done the best it can with what you've given it! That's great, right? The problem is that all of the minor compensations your body made because it didn't receive the nutrients it needs are not good. They create a cascading state of imbalance, deficiency and 'disease' within your body. It is a man-made imbalance created by your conscious choices. This imbalance lasts for years in most people. Then they wonder why they are gaining weight, losing energy, looking old, experiencing more pain, going through mood swings, generally feeling bad, getting wrinkles or gray hair—even though they may be exercising and eating a healthy diet and following all the latest "health rules".

Another way to think about the 100 buckets is to imagine there is a hole in the bottom of each bucket. As long as there is enough of the appropriate nutrient in each bucket, the hole remains plugged up and your energy, youthfulness, health, longevity, vitality and life force remain in balance. But, if you don't have enough of each nutrient in the appropriate bucket, all of these goodies simply leak out through the hole, thereby decreasing them. This, obviously, is not what you want to happen. That's why you want to keep all of the 100 nutrient buckets full at all times.

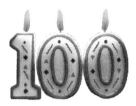

The Root Cause

In my 20+ years of research and according to the research and experience of a growing number of highly experienced physicians and natural health experts who have helped many patients achieve their ideal weight and eliminate disease simply by providing the body with the required spectrum of nutrients, the lack of the full spectrum of approximately 100 nutrients I just discussed is the only common sense root cause of obesity and the foundation for virtually all diseases. Of course many great minds have come to this conclusion; I simply learned it from them! You will read more about their thoughts on this subject in a coming chapter.

It just makes common sense, doesn't it? Nothing I have ever read in over 20 years of research makes more sense. Everything starts at the cellular level with nutrients and DNA. The nutrients your cells receive determine how efficiently and effectively your cells, DNA and bodily functions are able to perform their jobs.

The imbalances can affect not only your physical body at

every level, including hormones and brain chemistry, but also every level of your emotional, mental and psychological well being. Nothing in your total being is left untouched by nutrients. *Your body runs on nutrients,* and there's just no denying it. This is why experts believe that virtually all diseases should not even exist in the first place.

Joel Fuhrman, M.D., in his book *Eat To Live* states "Never forget, 99 percent of your genes are programmed to keep you healthy. The problem is that we never let them do their job. My clinical experience over the past twenty years has shown me that almost all of the major illnesses that plague Americans are reversible with aggressive nutritional changes designed to undo the damage caused by years of eating a disease-causing diet. The so-called balanced diet that most Americans eat causes the diseases Americans get."

Marie-France Muller, M.D., in her wonderful book about trace minerals called *Colloidal Minerals and Trace Elements*, refers to the "smallness" of this first step of receiving the spectrum of nutrients in a chapter titled "In The Kingdom Of The Infinitely Small." She states: "This level of our body's operation is one of life's smallest kingdoms. Here in this domain, it is not quantity that counts as much as a complete and balanced intake of all the minerals we need—as well as their quality and ability to absorb them easily."

So how can the lack of these nutrients create imbalances and disease? It's simple. It happens at the very beginning, at the smallest level. Your cells and DNA are missing something, so each step along the way your body compensates. Each compensation leads to another often greater compensation. It's like when you aim an arrow at a target that is 50 yards away. If you release the arrow just one or two degrees off course, by the time it travels 50 yards, you might miss the bull's-eye by 20 feet. Getting the first step wrong *magnifies and compounds* all the other compensatory steps along the way. Things get out of balance and you experience those imbalances as symptoms of the problem, including aches, pains, disease, weight gain, sleep problems, premature aging, lack of energy, etc.

It's common sense to get all your nutrients first, but it's certainly not common practice in America. And, now we're all paying the heavy price with our ultra-expensive and poor-outcome healthcare system.

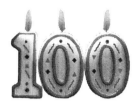

Is There Any Other Probable Common Sense Cause?

Quite a few natural health experts and medical doctors know, from their own research and patient use, that the lack of micronutrients is the root cause. You can read about their experiences in their books or websites if you are a disbeliever. Here are just a few of them:

- Dr. Weston A Price: *Nutrition And Physical Degeneration*

- Dr. Joel Wallach and Ma Lan, M.D.: *Rare Earths Forbidden Cures*

- Dr. Linus Pauling, two time Nobel Prize winner "You can trace every sickness, every disease and every ailment to a mineral deficiency"

- Max Gerson, M.D. founder of The Gerson Institute

- Gary Price Todd, M.D.: *Nutrition, Health & Disease*

- Joseph Mercola, M.D. www.mercola.com

- Joel Furhrman, M.D.: *Eat To Live*

- Bruce Fife, N.D.: *Eat Fat Look Thin*

- Marie-France Muller, M.D.: *Colloidal Minerals and Trace Elements*

I could go on and on, but I think you get the point. It's really just common sense. I discuss this in more detail in a later chapter.

Second, as Americans we know for sure that we are not suffering from a lack of:

- Water

- Calories from macronutrients

We may not be getting the right kinds of carbohydrates or fats and I will address that in the Nourish section of this book. But even if we were, we would still be severely lacking in the basic spectrum of 100 nutrients because the largest component of the 100, the full spectrum of trace minerals, are severely depleted from the soil.

Third, if you're still not convinced it could be this simple—that getting the full spectrum of micronutrients is the answer; the absolute root cause—then we can look at a diagnosis-by-exclusion example to remove any possible doubt. There are all types of beliefs and theories in the health, diet and nutrition fields about what the root cause really is. Some say that the pH of your body is the key. Others believe that eating foods low on the glycemic index is key. Still others say that antioxidants are the key. I have tried to address all of them below to show that only missing 100+ nutrients can be the true root cause:

- Is it possible to receive plenty of calories and still be severely nutrient deficient? Yes. This is America's problem today.

- Is it possible to be perfectly hydrated and still be severely nutrient deficient? Yes.

- Is it possible to obtain the optimal ratios of macronutrients, fat, protein, and carbohydrates and still be severely nutrient deficient? Yes.

- Is it possible to perfectly combine the right foods and still be severely nutrient deficient? Yes.

- Is it possible to consume many different pharmaceutical products or no pharmaceutical products at all and still be severely nutrient deficient? Yes.

- Is it possible to have a perfectly cleansed colon and a toxin free body and still be severely nutrient deficient? Yes.

- It is possible to have perfect hormonal levels, or to even take bioidentical hormones and still be severely nutrient deficient? Yes.

- Can you receive plenty of enzymes or probiotics from supplements and still be severely nutrient deficient? Yes.

- Is it possible to receive plenty of antioxidants and still be severely nutrient deficient? Yes.

- Is it possible to receive plenty of electrolytes and

still be severely nutrient deficient? Yes.

- Is it possible to receive plenty of fiber in your diet and still be severely nutrient deficient? Yes.

- Is it possible to drink plenty of herbal products, teas or exotic juices and still be severely nutrient deficient? Yes.

- Is it possible to exercise until you are thin as a rail or as lean and "ripped" as a body builder and still be severely nutrient deficient? Yes.

- Is it possible to have the world's strongest willpower or self control and still be severely nutrient deficient? Yes.

- It is possible to have an alkaline (vs. acidic) body pH and still be severely nutrient deficient? Yes.

- Is it possible to eat mostly low glycemic index (GI) foods, have perfect insulin and glucose control and still be severely nutrient deficient? Yes.

- Is it possible to have the perfect inner ecosystem and gastrointestinal health and still be severely nutrient deficient? Yes.

- Is it possible to be highly oxygenated and still be severely nutrient deficient? Yes.

- Is it possible to have very low stress levels and still be severely nutrient deficient? Yes.

- Is it possible to have perfect genetics and still be severely nutrient deficient? Yes.

- Is it possible to eat a 100% plant based diet, a 100% non-plant based diet or a combination of the two and still be severely nutrient deficient? Yes.

- Is it possible to have perfect mind control or visualization and guided imagery abilities and still be severely nutrient deficient? Yes.

What's left? Have I missed anything from all the popular health or diet books on the market? While all of the above things may be important, they are not a substitute for getting the full foundation of 100+ nutrients. Think about it. What else could possibly be the root cause—other than a deficiency of essential and trace nutrients your body needs but can't make? *Your body runs on nutrients* and there's just no denying it.

There is no other probable common sense cause. I have never come across a more logical, sensible cause in all of my years of research. The full spectrum of nutrients are the absolute foundation of everything else. We will review this again in more detail in a later chapter.

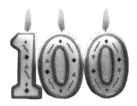

There Is No Substitute

There is no substitute for getting all 100+ of your micronutrients first every day! None.

Herbs aren't nutrients; they're more similar to medicines. And, you can't fake your body into not needing Vitamin B12 or Boron or Selenium or Vanadium or Linoleic Acid. You just can't. That's why getting your full spectrum of 100+ nutrients daily is the absolute foundation for everything! Getting a higher dosage of one or more nutrients does not compensate for a deficiency of three, seven, 10 or 50 other nutrients. For example, taking mega doses of Vitamin C or B12 does not eliminate your body's need for the full spectrum of 70+ essential and trace minerals or Vitamin K or D.

You also don't need specific products that claim things like "hair and nail support" or "flat tummy support" or "immune system support" or "nervous system support" or any other such claim. It's all just marketing hype. Nutrients don't just support those areas. What you put in your body affects every cell in your body. All you really need are your

100+ nutrients as they support *everything* in your body. They are the foundation that literally *everything* else rests on! They are the true starting point.

You can't fool your body; it needs what it needs and there is no substitute. Your goal is to flood your body with nutrients every day—but not just any nutrients—the full spectrum of 100+ essential and trace nutrients I've listed in this book.

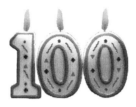

Food Pyramid Problems

Contrary to what you've been told your entire life, experts believe you cannot get all of your nutrients through the government recommended food pyramid. Health experts say the single belief that's been drilled into our heads since grade school of "You can get everything you need by eating according to the food pyramid" has been the source of more death and disease than from any other source. Even if you eat a pristine diet of the absolute freshest organic fruits and vegetables and grass fed meats, experts say you cannot receive the full spectrum of 100 nutrients today solely from food because many of these nutrients (especially minerals) are no longer in the soil.

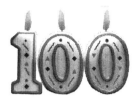

The Root Cause
Of Obesity

Progressive natural health experts now understand that obesity is not caused by a condition of excess. Rather it's caused by a deficiency—a deficiency of micronutrients. The symptom of this deficiency is an excessive and unnatural intake of calories as your body keeps you hungry in search of those missing nutrients. The nutrient deficiency is what keeps you eating and overeating, not your lack of willpower. The deficiency is what's causing your stress eating, binge eating and your resorting to food as a coping and comfort mechanism. Stress uses up a lot of nutrients! Yet, virtually every weight loss program on the planet teaches you that obesity is a disease of excess and is simply a formula of calories in minus calories out. No wonder it's said that 85% of people gain back all the weight they lost and then some within just a few years. They're solving the wrong problem and it's not the root problem. So, the symptom of the problem keeps coming back—the weight. You must solve the root nutrient deficiency problem to be successful.

Does this automatically mean that all skinny or lean people are getting their 100+ nutrients? No. That's a logical question since the lack of nutrients is believed to be the root cause of overeating and weight gain, therefore you might conclude if someone is able to control their appetite they must have all their nutrient buckets full, right? An estimated 95% of all people are said to be lacking in the full spectrum of nutrients—many of them are overweight and many are not. Many skinny or lean people get sick and die before age 100, or for that matter, before couch potatoes. Just because you're thin or lean doesn't mean you're healthy. Some people just have super metabolisms where they can eat whatever they want and they burn it off. I have friends that fall into this category. Other people are so busy they just don't get hungry. Others have willpower of steel. Still others have digestive disorders or discomfort and eating is a burden for them. Others may not handle stress well and just don't get hungry. Some work out a lot and this shuts down their hunger. There are a lot of reasons people can be thin or lean while still not obtaining their nutrients. But, just because these people are thin or lean does not mean they are healthier than you or will live longer than you. People who are thin or lean would still want to get all of their nutrients to achieve the other two goals of this book—health and longevity. People who are overweight would want to get all their nutrients for all three goals of this book—to become lean, healthy and longer lived.

I hope what I'm saying here does not sound too farfetched for you to believe. As stated earlier, we've been hearing for years in the media how Americans are the most overfed yet under-nourished or malnourished people on the planet! I just explained above exactly what that really means and why it's critically important to solve. It is the only logical root cause of America's health and weight problems.

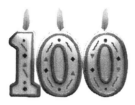

Doesn't Any Agency Monitor These Levels?

The governments of some countries have gone to great lengths to monitor the depletion of the nutrients in their soil and foods. Even the U.S. government has been monitoring the levels of 27 nutrients since 1909. You can review this long report at http://www.cnpp.usda.gov/publications/foodsupply/FoodSupply1909-2004Report.pdf.

The problem is that they are only tracking 27 of the approximately 100 nutrients experts say we all need every day. And they are not tracking the nutrients that are the absolute foundation of everything—the full spectrum of trace minerals. You can learn much more about nutrient depletion levels throughout the world in some of the books I've listed in the Resources section. There's just so much information available on this subject that I can't cover everything here.

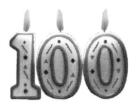

The Details Of
The 100 Buckets

Listed on the following pages are the approximately 100 essential and trace nutrients health experts say you need each day. I don't show the government's Recommended Daily Allowance (RDA) in the table, but I do show them in a separate table obtained from the government's official source. That way, you can visit the source directly as the numbers periodically change. The most current updated RDA's and daily values are located at the Food and Nutrition Information Center on the USDA website. Click on the first link called Dietary Reference Intakes: *Recommended Intakes For Individuals*. There's lots of other useful information on this page you may wish to explore, that's why I didn't just provide the single link.

Remember that the RDA is not the optimal dosage for the human body—it's simply the average dosage required by 98% of the healthy people of a certain gender and age group for all conditions so a deficiency does not occur. The optimal dosage may be much higher. Most supplement formulas contain a much higher dosage than the RDA. The RDA for the same nutrient also often varies by gender and age. A man often requires more than a woman for the same age group and a man and woman often require more than a child.

How You Can Obtain Them

The ideal way to obtain your nutrients is always from food first. That's because food contains many beneficial components other than essential and trace nutrients including enzymes, phytonutrients, nutrient cofactors, fiber, antioxidants and water. However, in a later chapter, I explain why experts believe getting all your nutrients from food is difficult today.

Over the years I have heavily experimented with many products and formulas in an effort to obtain all the essential and trace nutrients. At one point I was taking five different supplements and spending a lot of money to obtain them all. My family now takes no more than three supplements that contain all the nutrients we need. However, I am searching for a company that can create a high quality, low cost single product that contains just the nutrients I discuss in this book. I believe the key price point needs to be under $20 for a one month supply so every family can afford it. If you register on my website, I will keep you alerted to my progress.

How Much Do You Need?

Vitamins:
The government currently deems 14 vitamins as essential in their interactive website at http://fnic.nal.usda.gov/interactiveDRI/. The *ideal* list below contains 16 vitamins, one of which is bioflavonoids. It no longer is considered a vitamin, but used to be referred to as Vitamin P. The other

missing vitamin is Inositol but it is in most every supplement I have ever seen. The RDA for the vitamin dosages are listed at the link provided above. A good vitamin supplement should provide all of these.

Vitamins			
Vitamin A (Palminate)	Vitamin B (Thiamine)	Vitamin B2 (Riboflavine)	Vitamin B3 (Niacin)
Vitamin B5 (Pantothenic Acid)	Vitamin B6 (Pyridoxine)	Vitamin B12 (Cobalamin)	"Vitamin P" (Bioflavonoids)
Vitamin D	Vitamin E	Vitamin K	Vitamin C
Biotin	Choline	Folic Acid	Inositol

Minerals:
Mineral and trace mineral products vary in the number of minerals they contain. Products are usually assayed regularly to determine the average number of minerals in the product. I prefer an average of at least 70 minerals. They are:

- *Six Major Minerals:* These are stored in large volume in the body and include: Sodium, Chloride, Potassium, Calcium, Magnesium and Phosphorus. These will have individual dosage levels listed in a supplement.

- *Eight Essential Trace Minerals:* Chromium, Copper, Iodine, Iron, Manganese, Molybdenum, Selenium, Zinc. These will have individual dosage levels listed in a supplement.

- *56+ Additional Trace Minerals and Elements (not recognized as essential by the government):* The products my family takes usually contain at least 70 plant derived trace minerals. So, 56 or more of these minerals fall into this category. The government has not proven that these additional 56+ trace minerals are required by the human body. That also means that their value to the human body has not been *unproven* either. If scientists can't yet explain how something as uncomplicated as a maple tree can grow from such a tiny seed, how in the world will they ever be able to explain how 56+ minerals, required in microscopic dosages, effect the human body? It's impossible. That's why we simply need to resort to *common sense*. These minerals exist in the ocean and obviously were in the soil at one time. Many of these minerals have been depleted from the soil yet we still need them. So doesn't it make sense that we should simply obtain them in any way possible? The 14 minerals in the previous two categories can be found in most traditional vitamin or mineral supplements. However, trace minerals typically are not. Trace minerals will also not have individual nutrient dosage levels listed as their requirement, although critical, is very small.

- Dosage: The rule of thumb I was taught to follow is to take 600 milligrams of trace minerals (in liquid, powder or capsule form) for every 100 pounds of body weight.

- Try to obtain these minerals in a liquid, loose powder or powder in capsule form to maximize absorption.

- The best sources are usually from fruits and vegetables and to a lesser extent beans, nuts and seeds. Unfortunately, many experts believe trace nutrients and elements have been severely depleted from the soil and indicate no more than 20 are present in the soil due to modern farming practices. But, you must eat a highly varied, healthy diet in order to even come close to obtaining those 20. You will learn more about this in a later chapter.

RDAs for the 14 major minerals and essential trace minerals can be found at the government interactive link at http://fnic.nal.usda.gov/interactiveDRI/.

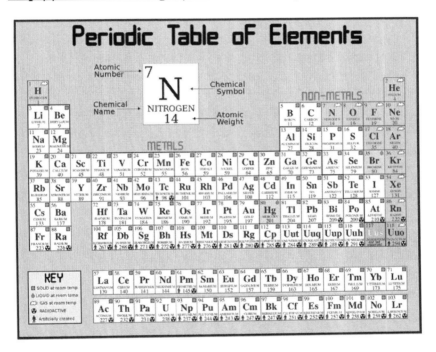

Nutritional minerals in foods are called elements, also known as atoms. You can find them among the 118 elements in the Periodic Table. The list of six major minerals and eight essential trace minerals are also in the Periodic Table.

Most of the mineral products I have taken over the years have contained a total of 50 or more minerals, trace minerals and elements. Some contain 54, others 60, others 72 or 75 minerals and elements. The number of minerals and elements in a product seems to be directly related to the source of the minerals. The sources of minerals will be discussed in a later chapter.

Because of this, I don't spell out in this book a specific list of trace minerals as the common belief seems to be "the more minerals the better". (The only place I have ever seen a specific number of minerals detailed is in Dr. Joel Wallach's book *Rare Earths Forbidden Cures*. He specifically lists and describes 60 minerals and trace elements that he believes are essential. He is a true pioneer in the area of *essential nutrients* and every effort should be made to read his book). Even minerals taken from the same location will vary in the number of minerals that are present at any given time. Sometimes a formula that quotes 70 minerals may in fact actually contain 67 – 72 minerals as conditions vary at the source. I presume that other health experts probably used Dr. Wallach's recommendations as a baseline and feel "the more minerals the better". You will have to choose what you believe is right for you. When possible my family usually aims for as many plant based minerals and elements as we can find in a supplement. Prices vary wildly among supplement companies and just because a product contains more minerals does not necessarily mean it will cost more. You can see our recommendation(s) in the Resources section.

Amino Acids:
Of the 12 amino acids listed in the table eight of them are currently considered essential by the government. Two of them are difficult to find in a supplement due to confusion caused by various entities over the years.

One of these is Tryptophan. Fortunately, there are a wide variety of foods that are good sources of Tryptophan and turkey is probably the most well-known source. Other foods high in Tryptophan are: chicken, beef, brown rice, nuts, fish, milk, eggs, cheese, fruit, vegetables and pumpkin seeds.

The other is Phenylalanine. Good dietary sources include protein-rich foods such as milk, meat, fish, cheese and soybeans (and also products that contain aspartame, which we don't use). Brewers yeast is a good source of most amino acids as well. A good supplement should contain at minimum 150 milligrams, in total, of the amino acids listed in the table.

Amino Acids			
Valine	Lysine	Threonine	Leucine
Isoleucine	Tryptophan	Phenylalanine	Methionine
Tyrosine**	Taurine*	Arginine*	Histadine*
*Not considered essential but believed to be important for developing children as well as adults. **Not considered essential as Phenylalanine can covert to Tyrosine.			

Essential Fatty Acids (EFAs):
Of the three essential fatty acids two of them—Linolenic Acid and Linoleic Acid—must come from your diet as they are truly essential. The third one, Arachidonic Acid, is considered essential only if you are deficient in Linoleic Acid. Recommended dosage of EFAs is usually stated as one to three teaspoons each day if taken in liquid form.

Good sources of Linolenic Acid are: canola oil, soybeans, walnuts, flaxseed, chia or hemp.

Good sources of Linoleic Acid are: pumpkin seeds, safflower oil, hemp oil, corn oil, walnut oil, peanut oil, sesame oil.

Essential Fatty Acids		
Linoleic (Omega 6)	Linolenic (Omega 3)	Arachidonic* (Omega 6)
*It only becomes essential if there is a deficiency of Linoleic Acid. You obtain it directly from dietary sources like meat, eggs, lard or dairy.		

Food Labels

Since these nutrients often appear on food labels, it is important you know how to read a food label. You can learn how to read a food label on the FDA's website.

Below are the amounts of the Daily Values (or DV which is similar to RDA) of macronutrients and micronutrients that are used when calculating all those percentages you see on food labels. Please note there are only 27 vitamins and minerals that are part of the daily value calculations. (Experts say we need approximately 100 nutrients in total, as you have learned.) Additionally, these values are based on a total caloric intake of 1,985 calories per day calculated as follows:

- Total Carbohydrate grams of 300 per day x four calories/gram = 1,200 calories (60% of total calories)

- Total Protein grams of 50 per day x four calories/gram = 200 calories (10% of total calories)

- Total Fat grams of 65 per day x nine calories/gram = 585 calories. (30% of total calories)

- Total Calories = 1,985 (100% of calories)

Be advised that there appears to be some confusion about

the number of nutrients the government deems essential. The current food label lists 14 minerals and 13 vitamins as essential or 27 nutrients in total. Yet, a current interactive government site located at http://fnic.nal.usda.gov/interactiveDRI/ lists 14 vitamins and 15 minerals or 29 nutrients in total as being essential. I just wanted to make you aware of it so you don't think it's a typographical error.

Daily Values (DV) Used for Food Labels

Nutrient	Amount	Nutrient	Amount
Biotin	300 mcg	Vitamin A	5,000 IU
Calcium	1,000 mg	Vitamin B-12	6 mcg
Chloride	3,400 mg	Vitamin B-6	2 mg
Chromium	120 mcg	Vitamin C	60 mg
Copper	2 mg	Vitamin D	400 IU
Folic acid	400 mcg	Vitamin E	30 IU
Iodine	150 mcg	Vitamin K	80 mcg
Iron	18 mg	Zinc	15 mg
Magnesium	400 mg	Total fat	65 g
Manganese	2 mg	Saturated fat	20 g
Molybdenum	75 mcg	Cholesterol	300 mg
Niacin	20 mg	Total carbohydrate	300 g
Pantothenic acid	10 mg	Fiber	25 g
Phosphorus	1,000 mg	Sodium	2,400 mg
Riboflavin	1.7 mg	Potassium	3,500 mg
Selenium	70 mcg	Protein	50 g
Thiamin	1.5 mg		

Mg = milligrams, mcg = micrograms, IU = international units

Source: Center for Food Safety and Applied Nutrition, 2002; National Academy of Sciences

The Only Pyramid
You Need To Know

We're all familiar with the food pyramid. It's tells you the number of servings of certain types of foods you should eat each day to supposedly receive all the nutrients you need to stay healthy, lean and long-lived. Healthcare experts say the food pyramid is invalid today because it's impossible to obtain the spectrum of the 100+ nutrients your body needs due to the nutrient depletion of our soils and our nutrient-poor, modern food supply. They believe you literally could not eat enough food in each category to obtain all the nutrients you need.

To solve this problem, below is something I created called The Essential And Trace Nutrients Pyramid (EAT Nutrients Pyramid[sm]). I believe this pyramid is the key to health, leanness and longevity because:

- Americans already receive too many calories and not enough nutrients. Nutrients are the foundation for every process in your body. The EAT Nutrients Pyramid focuses on getting your essential and trace nutrients first and on calories second. People don't get sick, fat and die prematurely due to a lack of calories, but rather due to a lack of nutrients. Once you get your nutrients you'll naturally eat fewer calories because there is absolutely no reason to overeat.

- Scientists around the world agree that calorie restriction while still getting all of your nutrients is the only scientific and proven approach to living longer. The EAT Nutrients Pyramid supports their findings because low levels of nutrients equate to higher caloric intake while high levels of nutrients equate to lower caloric intake. It's not really about calories in minus calories out. Rather, it's about the fact that the number of nutrients you receive determines the number of calories burned via your metabolism.

- I believe The EAT Nutrients Pyramid is the key

to eliminating child obesity, behavior problems in schools, bullying, many diseases and America's weight issue. It's easy and inexpensive, too.

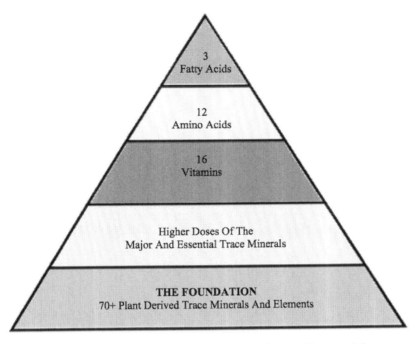

The Essential And Trace Nutrients Pyramid
(EAT Nutrients Pyramid[sm])

The Nutrient Imbalance Seesaw Effect[sm]

I want to illustrate the power of the 100+ essential and trace nutrients in another way to make sure you understand that they are the absolute foundation for everything that happens in your body. Everything begins with these nutrients. They are the first step of every process—that's why you want to get them first.

There is a constant trade-off taking place between your nutrient levels and your weight and health. I call this

The Nutrient Imbalance Seesaw Effect^{sm} or NISE^{sm}.

It's NISE^{sm} to get all your nutrients first!

As the first seesaw shows, not getting your 100+ nutrients will result in a higher caloric intake and more imbalances. The bottom seesaw shows that getting your 100+ nutrients will result in a lower caloric intake and fewer imbalances. If you can keep these images locked in your mind it may help you make healthier choices.

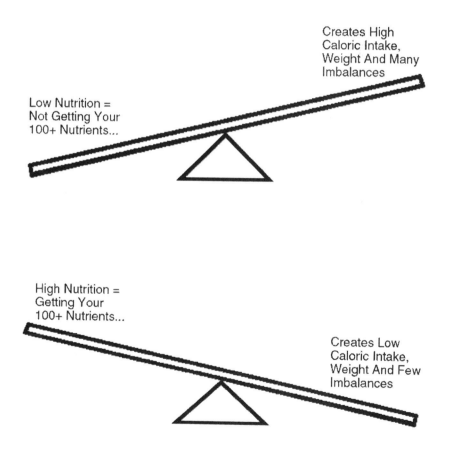

Solving Your Issues Always Begins "Here"

We've been hearing for years that Americans are the most overfed yet undernourished people on the planet. We've heard for years in milk, yogurt, cereal and other food and beverage commercials that most Americans are "missing important essential nutrients." Yet, nobody ever explained to us *exactly* what that meant, what we're missing and why we really need them. The term "essential and trace nutrients" is tossed around in a way like we're all supposed to know, instinctively, exactly what it means.

Now you know exactly what it means. It means you need approximately 100 essential and trace nutrients each and every day. They are comprised of 16 vitamins, 12 amino acids, 3 essential fatty acids and 70 or more trace minerals and elements. And, you need them in the appropriate quantities.

Please understand that, unless your issue is an emergency or is life threatening, solving any of your health, wellness, aging or longevity issues *always* begins with the same step - by getting *all of the 100+ essential and trace nutrients first!* Your issues exist because your body is most likely out of balance and starving for the proper nutrition. Most, if not all, of your issues can most likely be resolved simply by providing your body with the full spectrum of 100+ nutrients it needs, each and every day. The lack of any combination of the 100+ nutrients is the most common sense reason you're experiencing your issues in the first place. Use nutrients first to resolve and eliminate issues like:

- Excess weight; pain; sleep issues; fatigue or energy issues; aging issues; bone density issues like osteoporosis; teeth or mouth issues; cold and flu viruses; life threatening diseases or chronic health conditions; headaches; physical addictions like smoking, alcoholism or drug use; hormonal or sexual issues; stress, concentration or focus issues; behavior issues like ADHD, ADD, OCD, SAD, mood disorders, depression, compulsions, addictions; anger management issues; high blood pressure or cholesterol issues; etc., etc., etc.

What I'm implying is that for *any* non life-threatening physical, mental or emotional health issues that a human being can experience, the *first* thing you should do is always get your 100+ nutrients. Chances are, if you were getting all your nutrients regularly, you may have prevented your issue from ever happening in the first place. If you're a firm believer that your doctor knows best and that pharmaceutical medications are the best choice for your situation, that's fine. Listen to your doctor and take your prescriptions, but *also* get your 100+ nutrients. Remember, your condition did *not* develop from your body's *lack* of a particular pharmaceutical product. Nine out of ten times that product is only going to treat the symptoms of what's ailing you and it will not solve the root problem. The root problem originated because your body *lacked* the nutrients it really needed in the first place. So, why in the world would you continue to *not* give your body what it really needs and then turnaround and simply treat the symptoms of your problem with pharmaceutical products for the rest of your life? It's lunacy. Give your body what it needs each and every day to resolve issues you have now *and* to prevent new issues from developing in the future.

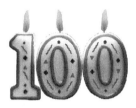

Why Empty
Buckets Are Bad

If you don't receive the full spectrum of 100+ nutrients daily, experts say it's bad for several vital reasons:

<u>You will dramatically increase your chances of gaining weight</u>. If you currently have a higher body fat percentage than is listed in the Lean Zone in the Body Fat Percent chart, you are eating too many calories. Your body is keeping you hungry even after you've eaten, hoping you will eat something that will provide the vital missing nutrients. You are consuming empty calorie foods, which is the formula for packing on the pounds. Additionally, experts say it is impossible for your metabolism to work optimally without the complete spectrum of the 100+ nutrients.

<u>These nutrients are the foundation for everything that happens in your body—everything!</u> These micronutrient raw materials represent the absolute foundation for *every* cell and process that occurs in your body and

mind. This includes how well your DNA and metabolism functions, whether your enzyme reactions work properly, how well your immune system functions, your brainpower and emotional stability, how well you deal with stress, how much you eat, how your body deals with pain, how efficiently your body burns fat and removes toxins, how fast your body heals, how well you age, how well you sleep, how well your digestive system functions, your energy levels, etc.

It is impossible for your body to function optimally in any area without the full spectrum of nutrients. Everything that happens in your mind or body relies on this complete micronutrient foundation. When I speak to people about this it's often hard for them to wrap their head around the fact that everything relating to how they look, feel, and perform begins with the full spectrum of 100+ nutrients. I mean, how can something so simple and basic be at the root of America's health and weight problems, right? Well, you could say the same thing about breathing. How can this invisible gas you inhale into your lungs be the life-giving force that it is? It seems like such a simple and basic process, right? But just try holding your breath and you can instantly see the effect it has on your body. It's the same with nutrients. You need oxygen, period. You need your spectrum of 100+ nutrients, period.

All *you* have to do is make sure you get *enough* oxygen. Your body already knows precisely what to do with it— once you have enough of it. It's the same with nutrients. You just need to make sure you're getting *enough of all of them*. Your body knows what to do from there. The only mistakes you can make are not getting all the nutrients you need or not getting them in sufficient quantity.

<u>Their deficiency is said to be the root cause of all disease states.</u> While experts agree that these nutrients, and especially the full spectrum of minerals, are the root of all problems in your body, at least one natural health expert believes that an average of 10 disease states can occur from each nutrient deficiency. So a deficiency of just one nutrient can increase your risk of acquiring 10 disease states; a deficiency of five nutrients can increase your risk of acquiring 50 disease states; a deficiency of 50 nutrients over time can increase your risk of acquiring 500 disease states! If there are only 20 minerals left in the soil and your body really needs 70 or more, you're missing 50 minerals and therefore are prone to 500 disease states...just by not getting your minerals! These aren't obscure, minor diseases that we've never heard of. They're the big ones like cancer, heart disease, stroke, arthritis, diabetes, depression and others. Although his predictions seem dire, they may actually be optimistic. For example, the mineral magnesium alone is said to regulate more than 300 critical reactions and body functions every day. It's so critical that low levels in your blood can lead to diabetes, heart disease, heart attacks and high blood pressure! What if every nutrient deficiency doesn't result in just an average of only 10 disease states, but 20, 30, 50 or more?

Here is a rather simplistic explanation of how the imbalances are believed to be created. Nutrients represent the absolute foundation—the bedrock—of all enzyme reactions in your body. The enzyme reaction is the actual first "spark" that begins all chain reactions at the cellular level. The belief is that each enzyme reaction that occurs in your body requires a specific combination of the 100+ nutrients as their fuel. Some reactions may require 10 nutrients. Others may require 30 nutrients while still others may require 40. If the required nutrients for a specific reaction are not available, the enzyme reaction either doesn't complete at all or it doesn't complete fully. All reactions from this point forward are therefore altered. These incomplete reactions are thought to be responsible for the imbalances that ultimately occur in the body.

Below, Marie-France Muller, M.D., in her book *Colloidal Minerals And Trace Elements*, discusses how the lack of nutrients alters DNA programming:

> Minerals play an essential role in the synthesis of DNA, the process of replication and duplication of cellular structures. In fact, the constant replacement of worn-out cells with new ones is entirely dependent upon trace elements (minerals). It is the body that determines what function a new cell will assume. The DNA molecule then programs it by providing it with genetic information in a way that ensures its proper functioning.
>
> When a cell has not been programmed well because of a deficiency of essential nutrients, it will simply continue to exist without fulfilling its proper role; the cell is alive but simply does not know what to do. The ramifications of this are not great when only a few isolated, improperly functioning cells are scattered here and there, but when they accumulate in a specific location, they may eventually form a tumor that could become cancerous. Or, when our bodies are no longer capable of consistently producing healthy cells, we may age prematurely or develop a number of diseases that could cause us to die before our time.

To me, this explains in very simple terms why cancer

could begin and spread. Why else would a perfectly normal cell randomly mutate and begin an unnatural replication process? Because its DNA has not been programmed properly. And why hasn't its DNA been programmed properly? Because it doesn't have the raw material essential nutrients it needs to properly program it.

Joel Fuhrman, M.D., in his book *Eat To Live*, states "Studies on both humans and animals have shown that plant-derived nutrients are able to prevent the occurrence of, and even reverse, DNA damage that may later result in cancer." Remember, everything in your body starts at the cellular and DNA level. If your body gets everything it needs at that initial level, you're stacking the odds heavily in your favor that everything else will automatically fall into place and remain in balance from that point forward.

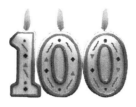

How To Easily
Fix Your Metabolism

People go to extreme lengths and expense to try to increase their metabolism so they burn more calories—endless aerobic or muscle building workouts, fat burners, protein powders, caffeine enhanced products, etc. All the while, an estimated 95 out of 100 of them are most likely deficient in the full spectrum of 100+ essential nutrients. They are taking all these difficult, costly steps to make themselves healthier yet they are missing the absolutely most simple and vital step that really matters. And, the step that would allow them to achieve their goals with much less effort.

These nutrients, especially the trace minerals, are the foundation to fixing your metabolism. I would highly recommend everyone read the amazing book by Marie-France Muller, M.D. called *Colloidal Minerals And Trace Elements*. It is one of the best books I have ever read on the need for the full spectrum of trace minerals and how their deficiency affects everything in the human body.

Here are just a few of the many quotes specifically about the benefits to your metabolism:

> "No cellular functions can be produced correctly if the body isn't receiving all the minerals and trace elements the metabolism needs...It so happens that all degenerative diseases originate, to one degree or another, [from] a severe mineral depletion of the body." - Dr. Robert La-Fave, United States Metabolic Research Center

> "Minerals and trace elements, essential to a healthy metabolism, have become even more precious because of the numerous deficiencies that are caused by the stresses and disruptions of modern life."

> "We know now that the minerals present in the plants we eat govern our cellular metabolism and are essential for maintaining good health and preventing disease."

The point is, there is no need to practically starve yourself, drain your bank account or push the limits of exercise until you nearly pass out just to get healthy and lean. The very first thing you must do is get your 100+ nutrients. Let that be your foundation. Let that do most of the "heavy lifting" for you. This step alone should reward you with at least 85% of the results you wish to achieve. And, it doesn't just help your metabolism, it helps your entire body. You want to work smarter, not harder. Working smarter means getting all of your nutrients first.

Remember, working hard to become lean doesn't mean you've become healthier or will live longer. It simply means you've become lean. You've only achieved one-third of the healthy, lean, longevity triangle.

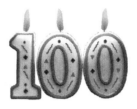

Stop Wasting Your Money

Many people are living their lives in a nutrient deficient state and don't know it. All they know is they don't look, feel, or perform the way they want to and they don't know why. They don't sleep well. They're tired. Their skin is dry or wrinkled. They weigh more than they want to and can't seem to lose weight because they're always hungry and eating and craving the wrong things. Their hair has turned prematurely gray. They feel emotionally unstable, stressed out and frustrated with life. This list goes on and on. As a result, in their desperation, they often "lunge" at all kinds of crazy quick-fix solutions. These include the latest celebrity diet books, infomercial products on TV, bizarre supplements, strange exercise equipment or workout routines, silly and often unhealthy diet programs, strange nutrient combinations, exotic herbal extracts or juices, fat burners, protein powders, etc.

All of this is done to try to relieve the symptoms created by their deficiency of the full spectrum of 100+ nutrients; the nutrients their body really needs—FIRST!

A person can waste thousands of dollars a year falling for these products and gimmicks. I was one of them until I learned what's in this book. All the while people have no idea that the most probable root cause of their issues is the missing spectrum of 100+ essential and trace nutrients. Their body is trying to compensate for this lack of nutrients and it's throwing them out of balance and creating symptoms or issues they don't like and don't know how to solve. It's like the old saying 'if you don't stand for something you'll fall for anything.' Make your stand for nutrients! You can't fool your body. **Get Your Nutrients First!**SM **Your body runs on nutrients and there's just no substitute for them.**

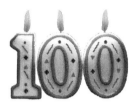

Marketers Prey On Desperate People

Many marketers take advantage of people in desperation. Here's an example from a recent experience. I was in a health food store talking to the cash register clerk about a product my wife uses. A woman around the age of 30 placed a product, that I've never seen before, on the counter. She walked away and I picked up the bottle to get a closer look and learned that it was an oil you take orally that claims to spot reduce belly fat (which is not possible of course). When she returned I asked her if she'd ever taken the product before and she said she had not. I asked her if she minded telling me about the goal she was trying to achieve with the product. She indicated that she wanted to reduce belly fat. This single product was selling for about $24, which was a one month supply. Out of curiosity, I asked her if she knew how many nutrients her body needs each day to achieve her ideal weight easily and inexpensively and for her metabolism to work optimally. She had the common response I hear all the time—"I have no idea." My point is, here she was willing to spend $24 on a *single* nutrient product claiming to do the impossible. Yet, for less than that, she could have received the full spectrum of 70+ minerals and trace nutrients that would have optimized her metabolism and strengthened her entire body.

Do you see the insanity in this? This is what I'm talking about how people fall prey to quick-fix claims that the advertisers know will persuade you in your moment of weakness! Many companies are getting rich and profiting from your confusion and desperation—while leaving you frustrated with poor results and less money in your bank account.

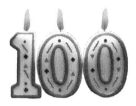

Inexpensive Insurance

Once you get your 100+ nutrients every day you've given your body the nutrient foundation it needs. You've heavily stacked the health, leanness, and longevity odds in your favor as much as possible. Your body is going to purr along as it was designed to do. You will sleep as you were designed to sleep. You will eat when you are hungry and will find it very difficult to overeat. You won't binge eat. Your metabolism will burn as hot as possible, just as it was naturally designed to do. Emotionally and mentally you will be more stable. Urges, compulsions or addictions will be reduced or eliminated. The way you handle stress will greatly improve. Your aches and pains will probably disappear. Everything works as it was designed to. How can you beat that for about the price of a few pizzas a month? I don't know of any cheaper insurance or solution on the planet, do you? No quick-fixes are needed once you get the foundational raw material of 100+ nutrients your body needs first every day. And if the economy and our wages continue to suffer while healthcare costs continue to skyrocket, everyone is going to need an easy and inexpensive solution to remain healthy.

It's silly and a total waste of your time and money to try anything else <u>until</u> you've gotten all your 100+ nutrients first for at least six months. I've thrown away shelves of supplements I used to take. Not only was I wasting a ton of money—I didn't feel nearly as good as I do now just taking my 100+ nutrients each day. Sometimes it can take six months for your nutrient buckets to fill up completely if you are seriously nutrient depleted, ill, or stressed. Once you fill your 100+ buckets, keep them filled by getting the proper nutrition each and every day.

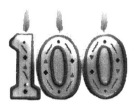

Would You Walk Around All Day Holding Your Breath?

If you were to walk around all day while holding your breath would you expect to look, feel and perform your best? Probably not. Yet, an estimated 95% of Americans are doing the equivalent of that nutritionally to their body and wondering why they don't look, feel or perform their best. Then, in an effort to look or feel better, they try all kinds of crazy quick-fix solutions like I mentioned earlier. Some of these "solutions" may appear to help a little, but nothing will provide the overall lasting effects they desire because they don't treat the root cause of the problem – the nutritional deficiencies.

If I tapped you on the shoulder and asked if you knew you were holding your breath and suggested you would feel better if you stopped holding your breath, what might you do? Would you say "no thanks, it can't be *that* simple—oxygen can't be *that* important?" Or would you thank me, inhale, and begin to feel better instantly?

The symptoms of not getting your nutrients every day may not appear as obvious as your constant need for oxygen, but it's just as dangerous in a more insidious way. When your oxygen supply is cut off there is no other way to obtain oxygen. That's why you notice the effects *immediately.* Yet, when you don't obtain the full spectrum of 100+ essential and trace nutrients you need each day, your body simply steals them from some other location inside your body, if they're available. Of course, the body is slowly weakening itself but remember, its primary goal is to keep you alive—not to insure structural integrity. That's why symptoms can occur slowly and can become chronic over time. Then you're diagnosed with a disease state and you wonder how this could have *suddenly just happened*? The truth is, in most cases, it probably took years for you to reach this state. Experts state that most of your health, weight and aging issues are caused from the simple error of not getting all your nutrients first.

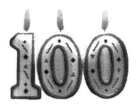

Upside Down Healthcare

Health experts estimate that 95% or more of us are deficient in the full spectrum of nutrients. That means 95% of us are not doing the absolute most basic step we need to do to keep our body healthy and lean easily and inexpensively—95% of us are 'holding our breath' and wondering why we don't feel or look the way we want to. Virtually all of your health, weight or aging issues are created from this one simple error.

When I used to restructure and turnaround companies years ago executives often used to make a common joke. As they contemplated fixing costly issues that should have been solved in the first place, they would say "We never have the time to do it right but we always make time to do it over." It's the same with healthcare. Because we don't do this tiny, little, inexpensive step right in the very beginning of getting all of our nutrients every day, trillions of dollars, heartache, pain, frustration and complexity are created to treat the symptoms of conditions that *shouldn't even exist in the first place.* It is really astonishing. An analogous quote for our healthcare might be "We never have the time to become healthy in the first place but we always make time for illness."

It's sad that people are dying and suffering because of this. Families are being torn apart unnecessarily. When my father and brother were dying in the hospital I used to spend quite a bit of time walking the halls talking to families and patients. It was heart wrenching to see children and adults dying as their families wept by their side, hoping for a miracle. It ripped my heart out and I never wanted that to happen again to my own family.

Please always remember—it's easier to stay well than to get well. My children walk around our home saying this when I point out something they should not be doing. "We know dad, it's easier to stay well than to get well." We also have this statement clearly posted in our exercise room. It really is easy to stay well when you understand how your body works and what it really needs.

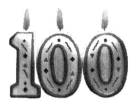

The Starting Point

So, shouldn't getting all of your nutrients every day be the absolute *first* place you turn to in order to solve your health, obesity, longevity, energy, sleep, aging, pain and other issues? Isn't that the simplest, least expensive and most common sense solution to our health and obesity woes as a country? Wouldn't brilliant thinkers like Albert Einstein have embraced this *first* if faced with the same problem—just making sure our entire population gets all of its nutrients every day? Conversely, if 95% or more of people were getting these nutrients every day and America *still* had all its weight and health problems only *then* we would have a very, very big problem on our hands and the current healthcare model in America might make some sense. I believe only then should we be doing what we are doing now as a country in regards to healthcare.

But as a country we've chosen to implement the most complex, destructive and expensive solution first without even making sure our citizens have covered the easy and inexpensive essentials and basics first. We're doing it all backwards and upside down. Everyone agrees America's current healthcare model is not effective or sustainable. That's why giving everyone health insurance or inventing new tests, drugs, and procedures will *not solve* the true root cause of our problems. It won't cure diabetes or cancer or heart disease. It just further increases healthcare costs and makes more money for the healthcare industry. It just prolongs the pain and agony of our country. As Winston Churchill is famous for saying "America always chooses the right option, but only after it's exhausted all other possible options." Let's fix the root reason people are getting fat and sick, first. Let's heavily stack the odds in people's favor first, before we do what we're doing now as a country. It is the only humane thing to do for every man, woman and child in our country.

Sure, it will require a transition from a disease care model to a preventative healthcare model, but we have no other option. Our current model is completely unsustainable and everyone knows it. Yet, no one seems to know what to do. What to do is easy if America chooses the most humane option—follow the advice from the experts in this book! Giving everyone in America the 100+ nutrients each and every day is the most humane and common sense method of healthcare on our planet.

How can the citizens of a country, where 90% of the food they eat is processed, be getting all their required nutrients? They can't – it's impossible and our bodies are screaming that loud and clear. If you were driving down the highway at 65 miles per hour and suddenly a wheel fell off, then smoke started coming out of your engine, then your dashboard caught on fire, then your steering wheel popped off...would you keep accelerating? Well, that's exactly what America's healthcare system is doing and everyone's standing around scratching their head wondering how to fix things. It's easy—just teach people what their body needs in the first place and help them get it.

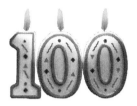

This Could Not Have Been The Original Healthcare Plan

The healthcare mess we're in wasn't the original plan (I hope). As people began getting fewer and fewer nutrients over the years, either through soil depletion or through eating more processed foods, naturally people began to get sicker and fatter. People from other countries who were once lean and healthy move to America and often gain 20 to 30 pounds, or more. I spoke with a family from another country recently who was complaining about this. It happened so gradually they said. I told them the fable about how to boil a frog. If you want to boil a frog, do you throw him in boiling water while he's still alive? No, he'll jump right out. But, if you place him in room temperature water and gradually increase the temperature, he will ultimately boil as he won't be able to sense the slight differences in temperature change. "Yes, yes" they said, "we're boiled frogs!"

Americans have been "boiling the frog" over the past 70 years and have slowly evolved to a state of obesity and poor health. It happened so gradually, but it can be turned around quickly!

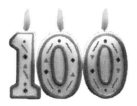

Animals Get These, Humans Get Health Insurance

Farmers must be smarter than the average human. They don't buy health insurance for their animals. They can't afford to. So, they *have to* practice preventative health to keep their animals healthy in the simplest and least expensive way possible so the prices you and I pay for our food remain reasonable. What if you were a farmer and had an entire herd of sick cattle and someone suggested that the herd may not be getting all the nutrients it needs. You then decided to give the entire herd all the nutrients it needs every day through a special new feed supplement you discovered. Don't you think at least half of the herd might respond well and become totally healthy over the next year?

Dr. Joel Wallach, in his book *Rare Earths, Forbidden Cures* talks about just this issue regarding problems in the American turkey industry one year. A majority of the birds were dying and it was later discovered they were suffering from a *single* nutrient deficiency. Once the birds were given that nutrient, none of them died the following year from that condition, not a single one, according to Dr. Wallach.

What works for animals will work for us. A cell is a cell. There's virtually no difference between what the cells of an animal or human need to stay healthy. Farm animals get everything they need in their farm feed. Every bite of feed contains the full spectrum of nutrients each species needs to remain healthy. Farmers are smart— they get it right from the start. That's because they want to keep costs low while keeping the health of their animals high. It will work just as well for humans.

That's why natural health experts say the moment a new patient enters a hospital in America, he or she should *immediately* be "prescribed" the appropriate dosage of the full spectrum of 100+ essential and trace nutrients each and every day. The lack of these nutrients is the reason why most of us end up in the hospital anyway, so if the goal is to heal us as quickly and inexpensively as possible, there's certainly no better way to do that than through providing these vital nutrients to patients.

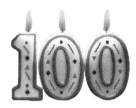

Incredible
Savings Are Possible

What if just half of our total population of roughly 340 million people could reduce that $7,400 per person healthcare cost to around $240 per person (about the cost of a year's supply of the full spectrum of 70+ minerals)?

That would be a savings of...

170 million people times roughly $7,000 a year savings (approximately $7,400 - $240)...or...

One trillion, one hundred ninety billion dollars each year! $1,190,000,000,000!

What if we decided only half this many people could save this much money, meaning only ¼ of our total population could virtually eliminate any healthcare requirements? That would be $595 billion in savings each year! $595,000,000,000!

What if we decided this was still too optimistic and we decided only half of that or 1/8 of our total population could virtually eliminate any healthcare requirements? That would be $298 billion in savings each year! $298,000,000,000!

Hard to believe, isn't it? All these savings are achieved from doing something so simple and inexpensive *right from the start*. This level of savings is achieved if just 12.5% (1/8) of America's population (about 42 million people) saved about $7,000 a year on out of pocket health spending simply by getting healthier. To put this $298 billion savings number in perspective, America's total 2012 military budget is $707 billion. It alone is always the largest part of America's annual spending. By doing something so ridiculously easy and inexpensive and by using common sense we can save the equivalent of about half of America's largest single cost by hardly even trying. And, this doesn't even include the productivity improvements in the workplace that would be realized from employees not becoming ill.

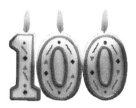

Houston We Have A Knowledge Problem

A few years ago when I finally came to understand the true power of getting all the 100+ nutrients each day, I struggled to believe what natural health experts said about 95% of our population not receiving these nutrients—or for that matter even knowing about them. So, over the past 14 months I did my own little unscientific test. I made it a point to ask at least 10 adults a month (most of whom I did not know) from all different walks of life and apparent income levels, education levels, and age groups a simple question:

Do you know how many nutrients experts say the human body needs each day to remain healthy, lean, and long-lived as easily and inexpensively as possible?

For the reader, remember that a correct answer would be in the ballpark of 100 nutrients. Guess how many people answered in that range? *None of them! Not a single one.* A few responded with answers like "nine" or "37" or "40" just as fun guesses, but most just laughed and responded "I have no idea." Yet, if you asked people what they breathe to stay alive, I'm guessing 100% of them would say "oxygen" or "air." I did not think to keep detailed statistics on this study as I was certain I was eventually going into run into a group of people who knew the answer. It never happened. Granted, approximately 140 people is not representative of our entire population. But, the fact that not a *single* person knew the nutrient foundation needed by their body is pretty scary indeed. That's why this information needs to be taught in schools beginning at an early age and why we need to get the word out.

Remember my little test. Perform it yourself on your friends and family now that you know the answer. See what kind of answers you get. I'm certain your results will (unfortunately) parallel mine.

We are talking about the most likely, common sense root causes of obesity and disease in America and in the world today, and the most common answer during my little test is "I don't know." Would it be safe to say "Houston, we have a knowledge problem!"? A very, very, very BIG problem? Maybe it's just so darn simple, basic, unglamorous, and mundane in a high-tech and sensationalized society that people don't even consider the thought of something like "nutrients" as having any real power. Isn't breathing mundane and boring too? Yet, what happens when you hold your breath? That's why you need to get your 100+ nutrients first! Everything, and I mean everything, begins at the cellular and DNA level. Give your cells and DNA what they need and you've created the essential foundation your body needs.

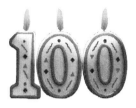

How To Eliminate Child Obesity

First Lady Michelle Obama has stated publicly that her number one goal while her husband is President is to eliminate childhood obesity. Below is a simple, inexpensive and common sense way for her to do it.

- Teach all children, starting in middle school, about the importance of the EAT Nutrients Pyramid[sm] that I outlined in an earlier chapter. Also teach them how their body works and how these nutrients are the foundation for every process in their body.

- Teach children to obtain their calories from fresh, whole foods. This can be done using the current food pyramid, although I would rearrange some of the categories.

- Provide an inexpensive, easy method for children to receive these nutrients as a backup plan (for example through supplementation). This is because children are going to be less likely to eat healthy than adults.

- As a further backup plan, absolutely mandate that all food and beverage manufacturers who sell products in schools fortify their products with the full spectrum of 70+ plant derived trace minerals, at minimum. That way, even if children choose snack foods over whole foods they will still be getting their necessary nutrients. (Remember, plant minerals are said to be nearly 100% absorbable, so they provide much greater value and more benefit at a lower cost—something all schools are concerned about today.) Every lunch served should contain the spectrum of nutrients as well.

- Continue with physical fitness programs as is currently done in schools.

The benefits of the above steps extend far beyond just eliminating childhood obesity. Students will be better behaved in class, will have more focus, will get better test scores and bullying should be reduced or eliminated. This is not a hunch. You can read about these beneficial 'side effects' in Dr. Wallach's book *Rare Earths Forbidden Cures*. Amazing things happen when the human body receives all the nutrients it needs. If the above points seem incredibly simple and easy—that's because they are! That's the whole point. It is easy and inexpensive. This is not rocket science. It's not complicated. Giving your body what it needs is just common sense.

Remember earlier when I told you how my wife had two consecutive miscarriages and how any further miscarriages were totally eliminated by her taking an inexpensive baby aspirin a day during her pregnancies? If our OB/GYN was not astute and practical he could have sent us both to the hospital or to specialists for many time consuming, expensive tests that may have cost $100,000 or more! But, he did the right thing at the right time—*at the very beginning*, and now we have our amazing children to thank him for.

The information in this book is equivalent to that single, simple, inexpensive baby aspirin given at the very beginning. It's not any more complicated than that. These nutrients can have the curative effects on your health, weight loss efforts, longevity and your children's health like the baby aspirin had on our miscarriages. You just need to *get the nutrients*. Just give your body what it needs in the first place and almost everything else will *automatically* fall into place—just the way it was designed to do.

If you find this hard to believe please make sure you read the books in the Resources section.

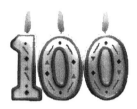

The Basics Of Getting What You Need

As stated earlier, experts state that 95% of people do not receive the entire spectrum of 100+ nutrients every day. Remember my own little survey of 140 people? None of them had any idea how many nutrients their body needed each day. Yet, surveys show that over 40% of Americans do take a multivitamin pill daily. People are trying to do what they *think* is right but they really don't know for sure what to do so they think about vitamins first. (At minimum they should be thinking about the 70+ trace minerals first.)

Keeping that in mind, there are several things you want to be certain of when you supplement. They are:

- You want to take the <u>right nutrients.</u> The 100+ essential and trace nutrients your body needs.

- You want to take these nutrients at the <u>correct dosage</u>.

- You want to take them in the <u>most absorbable form</u> (which is usually a liquid, or a powder that you add to a liquid).

- Ideally you want to take a supplement with nutrients that are as close to those found in <u>real food</u> as possible, not synthetic or man-made nutrients.

Without following these considerations you are wasting your money and more importantly, could be jeopardizing your health. Taking just certain nutrients is referred to as 'isolated' or 'fractionated' nutrition. Most people in America today do this…and marketers know they will fall for it. People see a commercial for something on TV or in a magazine, it sounds good, and they start taking that nutrient. But all the while, they're not even close to getting their full spectrum of 100+ raw material nutrients that represent the foundation for everything. More importantly they could be putting their body in an even greater state of imbalance or disease by fractionating their nutrition.

It's a favorite tactic of food, beverage or supplement marketers to prey on your confusion. They will often boast that they've added super nutrient XYZ to their formula and it decreases fat or increases muscle or whatever else they claim. Please remember there is no single magic nutrient that will do this. It's like saying you get the sound of an entire orchestra from just a single trumpet. It's impossible.

Here's another problem most people don't know about: Look at all the popular vitamin enhanced beverages on the market today. Millions are spent marketing these products to consumers. But, few if any of these products that I have seen contain the spectrum of minerals or anything close to the full spectrum of nutrition. That's unfortunate because experts say vitamins are essentially useless without minerals. If you're looking for these products to improve your health you may be just throwing your money away and potentially causing more problems—here's why. When you ingest only vitamins, your body doesn't automatically say "yippee, vitamins!" Your body looks at what you've ingested and has to decide what to do with it—keep it or excrete it. If it decides to keep it, it has to be able to metabolize those vitamins into a form that is absorbable. To metabolize vitamins you need minerals. If you are not taking minerals in, your body will have to pull those minerals out of your own body—from your bones or organs—to metabolize the vitamin. This is not what you want to happen as it can create further imbalances and potential disease. To counteract this you can add plant based minerals directly to these beverages.

Think of how nature provides nutrients in fresh, whole foods. No whole, fresh food provides only one nutrient or any single nutrient in mega doses. Whole foods contain multiple nutrients from multiple micronutrient groups in relatively small doses. They also contain enzymes, phytonutrients, fiber and nutrient co-factors that help break down and metabolize the nutrients.

"It's a false assumption that foods are good because of singular nutrients," says Roberta Anding, RD, spokeswoman for the American Dietetic Association (ADA) and dietitian for the National Football League's Houston Texans. "It's really the package deal that Mother Nature puts together [that matters]."

As you eat fresh, whole foods throughout the day (as

you are supposed to) you are getting a gentle trickle of the spectrum of nutrients your body needs and can easily absorb and utilize. And, more importantly, you are getting most everything you need to metabolize those nutrients without having to steal vital nutrients from your own bones or organs. Remember, your goal is to keep this process of getting healthy, lean, and long-lived as simple, inexpensive and common sense as possible. That's why I keep repeating myself about the need for the 100+ nutrients first. You want to make obtaining these nutrients the focus of how you eat each day. It is the first step everyone should follow.

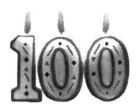

Why Doesn't Everyone Do This?

Experts estimate that 95% or more of people are not receiving their full spectrum of essential and trace nutrients every day. While writing this book I often wondered why everyone doesn't supplement. Here's what I came up with:

- They don't think they need to supplement because they believe they can get all their nutrients from their food supply or The Food Pyramid. They don't realize that no matter how much they eat, it is impossible for the average human to eat enough to obtain all their nutrients today.

- They don't know how to supplement. They're not sure what to do so they pop a cheap vitamin pill thinking that's all they need, not knowing it could actually be causing further imbalances in their body.

- They incorrectly believe that what they eat

doesn't have much of an effect on their health or that their health is determined primarily by their genetics.

- They're depressed and simply don't care about their health or about what happens to them.

- They perceive supplementing as an additional cost. Here's how to overcome that:

  - In my family we cut elsewhere to pay for supplements so we don't really incur any additional cost.

  - If you supplement properly you incur a net savings because you'll be saving on out-of-pocket healthcare costs and you'll be able to eliminate supplements you're taking now that probably aren't necessary once you receive your 100+ nutrients. Plus, when your body is properly nourished you will automatically eat less and therefore spend less on groceries.

  - If you tried to get all your 100+ nutrients from your food supply you'd be spending a lot more money on groceries than on the supplements...and still not getting all the nutrients you need.

  - Simply cut a few alcoholic beverages each month or a few of your favorite fancy coffee beverages or one or two family dinners out and you've easily covered the cost of supplementation. There is no cheaper insurance than supplementation.

  - If you're not sick you won't suffer from lost wages and will actually earn more money.

• Your employer may pay more of your health insurance costs if you become leaner or healthier or don't get sick as much.

You now know that you really must supplement to obtain all of the nutrients your body needs in the proper dosages. You now know which nutrients you need. And, you now know that cost really is not an obstacle to supplementing. Give it a try and I think you will be amazed at the results.

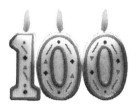

Why It's Difficult To Get Everything You Need

Below is a listing of some of the most common reasons you can stuff yourself with the healthiest and most carefully grown organic foods on the planet and still not receive the complete spectrum of 100+ essential and trace nutrients you need. Primarily, I am talking about the full spectrum of 70+ minerals below. Many of the other nutrients can be obtained, at least at some random dosage level, if you eat a healthy balanced diet. However, you will have no idea what nutrients are in your food or their dosage, as explained below.

1. <u>Minerals are not evenly disbursed throughout the soil</u>. Minerals run through the soil in vein-like formations. So if you plant 50 rows of corn the first three rows may be rich in one particular mineral. The next ten rows may be low in all minerals. The next seven rows may contain one or two minerals. Even the nutrients found in each ear of corn on the same

plant will most likely vary. So, it's totally by chance that you receive any nutrients or minerals at all. It's a highly random occurrence and you never know what you are getting.

2. <u>Modern farming methods deplete the soil</u>. Soils are much lower in nutrients, including minerals, than they were just 50 or 60 years ago. If you have any doubt please read Elmer Heinrich's book *The Untold Truth*. In approximately seven years soil becomes depleted of minerals if that same soil is farmed each year. Minerals aren't manufactured by the soil. Once they're gone they're gone forever unless they're added back in through acts of nature (like flooding) or by man in the form of fertilizer. Modern farmers only add three minerals to the soil, known as N-P-K (Nitrogen, Phosphorus, Potassium), which help to maximize crop yield per acre, not increase nutrient levels. Adding the entire spectrum of trace minerals back into the soil is supposedly too expensive and cost prohibitive. Remember, farmers don't receive bonuses for producing high nutrient foods. Then the chemicals and pesticides that are added to the soil destroy the vital, tiny microbes that are necessary to break down organic matter back into its mineral components. It's a losing battle because nutrients are removed from the soil, they're not added back in and the ability of the soil to regenerate is compromised. It's a lose-lose-lose situation.

I watched an entire one hour long TV show a few years ago about how scientists were trying to create the perfect tomato. "Perfect" to them meant brilliant color, nice size and long shelf life. *Not once* during the entire hour long show was the word "nutrient" mentioned.

Marie-France Muller points out in her book *Colloidal Minerals And Trace Elements* that organic farmers who cultivate their land through the use of natural fertilizers certainly avoid the disastrous problems that come with chemical fertilizers and dangerous pesticides. But, because cultivation of any kind depletes the minerals and nutrients in the soil and because plants do not have the ability to synthesize (make) minerals, ultimately the organic farmer's produce will not be any more nutritious than produce grown following standard commercial practice. Any soil under cultivation requires that its minerals and nutrients be restored regularly. There is an ongoing debate about whether organic produce has a significantly higher nutrient content than standard produce. I have seen studies that give a slight edge to organic produce. If you choose to eat organic produce the value appears to be reduced toxins from pesticides and not necessarily increased nutrition.

Fruits and vegetables get their taste primarily from minerals. The taste and sweetness of produce is measured in something called a BRIX value. A higher BRIX value means more robust flavor, which means there is a higher mineral content in that particular piece of produce. Bland tasting produce has a lower BRIX value. You can easily compare the taste of various brands of standard and organic produce to learn which has a more robust flavor. For example, a tomato at a local farm stand would hopefully have a more robust flavor than one purchased at a typical supermarket simply because it may have a few more minerals in it. I ate a tomato last week from a grocery store and although it looked fine, if I closed my eyes and was asked to identify what it was I would have had no idea. It was bland and tasteless.

An article in National Geographic, September 2008, titled *Scarce Fertility*, states "Today more than six billion people rely on food grown on just 11 percent of the global land surface. Even less ground – a scant 3 percent of the Earth's surface – offers inherently fertile soil." Soil degradation can transform productive zones into wastelands with tragic speed. "The history of every nation", U.S. President Franklin Roosevelt said, "is eventually written in the way in which it cares for its soil."

It's no wonder experts say you need to eat 10 or more servings of vegetables today to equal just one serving from 50 years ago. You can learn more about these facts in a book by Elmer Heinrich called *The Root Of All Disease*. His book also contains numerous studies from around the world showing the drastic reduction in the nutrient content of foods and soils over the past few decades.

3. <u>Erosion reduces topsoil</u>: Topsoil contains a majority of minerals that we want our food to contain. Unfortunately, over time, a good portion of topsoil can erode away from cultivation, strong winds or strong rains.

4. <u>Pesticides and chemicals added to soil deplete nutrients</u>. Pesticides not only pollute

our planet, they disrupt the natural bacteria, microbes and tiny creatures that live in the soil in an act that has been likened to sterilizing the soil. These vital bacteria and microbes help the plant root assimilate the nutrients that exist in the soil and without them, the plant can not take up all the nutrients that it should. Interestingly, for about the past four years, we have not used any fertilizer or pesticides in our own garden. We simply spray it with a diluted solution of trace minerals a few times in the early part of the growing season and we have no pests or insects at all. That's because once the plant receives all the trace minerals it needs through the soil, it is able to create its *own* pesticide due to a very strong immune system. If minerals can do this for plants, imagine what the spectrum of minerals will do for your own immune system!

5. <u>Processing of our foods removes nutrients</u>. Experts say 90% of what Americans eat is processed. Processing results in empty calories—all you get are calories and few to no nutrients. This keeps you hungry and eating. Your goal is to eat high nutrient foods with low calories. Many foods are fortified with a few minerals and vitamins, but they *should* be fortified with the full spectrum of trace minerals, at minimum. Ideally, our processed foods should contain the entire spectrum of 100+ essential and trace nutrients in every bite.

6. <u>Your consumption of sugar increases the depletion of nutrients from your body</u>. This is made worse by the fact that sugar consump-

tion per person in America is at an all time high. This means whatever nutrients you do receive can be rapidly excreted from your body if you eat a lot of sugar. In an earlier chapter I explained how I was suffering from severe cholesterol and triglyceride imbalances in my teens even though I was "ripped" and "looked" healthy. Experts have told me it was because I was chugging a gallon of extremely highly sugared iced tea each day after working out. And, I did this for years! Not only was I not eating healthy and not getting my nutrients, I was sweating out many nutrients each day and the sugar was further driving nutrients out of my body. I was also doing nothing to replenish these nutrients. I'm told I was severely nutrient and mineral depleted and this is the precise reason why experts believe athletes, and those people who exercise a lot, die suddenly and much younger than couch potatoes.

7. Transportation of foods reduces nutrients. Today our food comes from all over the world. Many foods today are picked green so they can ripen during the trip to your grocery store. They therefore don't contain the same level of nutrients that they would if left to ripen on the vine. Additionally, nutrients decrease after a two to five day plane, ship, train or truck ride. Nutrients also decrease while the foods sit on grocery store shelves.

8. Drinking too much water increases the depletion of nutrients, including minerals, from your body. There seems to be a belief in America that you have to be carrying a water bottle around all day long and sipping it constantly whether you're thirsty or not. Any nutrients

you do happen to get from your food can be *easily* washed away before they are absorbed due to excess water intake. Additionally, drinking a lot of water right before or with a meal to help you feel full can reduce nutrient absorption because they're more quickly excreted.

9. <u>Exercise increases the depletion of nutrients, including minerals, from your body</u>. When you exercise you sweat. Sweat is a "soup" of lots of things, including the spectrum of nutrients and minerals. If you sweat regularly and don't refill your 100+ nutrient buckets you are harming your body. Natural health experts believe this is the main reason people who exercise a lot, including professional athletes, die suddenly and much earlier than the average couch potato. It's not the exercise that kills them—it's the fact they are not replenishing the nutrients they sweat out and it creates dangerous imbalances in their body. If you sweat a lot you *must* replenish your 100+ nutrient buckets every day.

10. <u>Stress increases the depletion of nutrients in your body</u>. If you're alive today you're under stress. The state of the world, the state of the economy, the state of your personal finances due to the recent financial crisis, wars, raising a family, human tragedy, natural disasters and everything else in life depletes the supply of nutrients in your body because your body works much harder when it's under stress.

11. <u>Our toxic bodies use up more nutrients faster</u>. Our bodies contain hundreds of toxins from medicines and what we eat, breathe and

drink. Your body has to work much harder to neutralize and excrete these toxins and you guessed it—that uses up vital nutrient supplies much faster. Plus, if your intestines are coated with a toxic sludge of mucous and hardened feces (as most people's are), you will not be able to absorb nutrients properly.

12. <u>Fractionated nutrition can deplete nutrients in your body</u>. As I explained earlier, taking isolated nutrients—rather than the full spectrum of nutrients—forces your body to use up precious nutrients because the isolated nutrients have to be metabolized in some way before they can be absorbed.

13. <u>Genetic modification reduces nutrient content in hybrid fruits and vegetables</u>. Producers create genetic "hybrid" forms of fruits and vegetables not for increased nutrient content, but to make them last longer and look prettier to consumers. Hybrids often contain more water, sugar and supporting tissue so they have a longer shelf life. They look better, ship better and often weigh more (thereby costing you more), but contain very low nutrient content. For example, by the FDA's own admission, a popular hybrid form of broccoli contains 35% lower calcium and magnesium than other hybrids; hybrids themselves are 50% lower in calcium and magnesium than normal broccoli; and normal broccoli has less than half the calcium and magnesium than broccoli did in 1975.

14. <u>Alcohol consumption depletes nutrients in your body.</u> As your body metabolizes alcohol valuable nutrients are used in the process.

The above points create a scary scenario. We're not getting all the nutrients we need in the first place and we're depleting the nutrients we do receive faster than ever before. And, we're not even absorbing them in the first place. America is now witnessing the effects of this dangerous and deadly combination in our obesity rates, chronic health and aging problems and skyrocketing healthcare premiums.

Your body is incredibly wise. Your body *never* "turns" on you and is always trying to do the best it can with what you've provided it. If it has to make a choice between keeping you alive or maintaining its own structural integrity—it will choose life. That's why you see people walking around who are alive but have very weak or frail skeletal structures, are hunched over, get sick all the time, have terribly wrinkled skin, etc. Their body is choosing to keep them alive but it has to rob nutrients from bones, organs or body parts to do that. Robbing those areas of nutrients creates all kinds of problems, imbalances and potential disease states. It's much easier to simply get all the nutrients you need every day in the first place. It really is that simple.

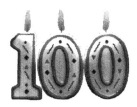

The Only "Proven" Approach To Life Extension

The fields of anti-aging and longevity are very interesting. Brilliant scientists from all over the world are independently researching this subject and are trying to find the Fountain Of Youth and the secrets to longevity. The only thing they've agreed upon so far is that calorie restriction, while still getting all your nutrients, can prolong human life up to 40%. Calorie restriction means you are consuming foods low in calories but rich in all the micronutrients. These types of foods are called *nutrient dense* foods. If scientists agree that you can prolong your life up to 40% through a calorie restricted diet and the average lifespan in America is currently 78.2 years, then adding 40% to that adds another 31.2 years for a total lifespan potential of 109.4 years. That's pretty close to how long scientists believe the typical human lifespan should be.

So why is calorie restriction while obtaining all your nutrients so vital to living longer? Digestion is said to be the biggest stressor on the human body. Low calorie, high nutrient foods are usually very easy to digest so they put very little stress on your digestive system and body. Your body produces two major types of enzymes: digestive enzymes and metabolic enzymes. Digestive enzymes help digest your food. Metabolic enzymes do the majority of repairing and healing in your body. Enzyme pioneers like Dr. Edward Howell believed that your body has a limited ability to produce enzymes. He believed that if your body is busy producing digestive enzymes to digest food that is dead (contains no live enzymes because it was heated), it will not be able to produce enough healing metabolic enzymes. On the other hand, if you are eating live foods that contain the enzymes necessary to digest the food you've just eaten, then you will have an abundance of metabolic enzymes available to heal and repair your body.

As the theory relates to calorie restriction, if you eat fewer calories from heated foods your body will have to make fewer digestive enzymes and will therefore have an abundant supply of metabolic enzymes available for repairs and healing. A body that is repairing itself faster than it is breaking down will naturally live longer. With calorie restriction the belief is that you are doing very little to stress or tear-down your body and you are getting all your nutrients and enzymes necessary to constantly repair your body.

If you recall from an earlier chapter, the definition of aging is when "your body breaks down faster than it can rebuild itself." You can therefore see why calorie restrictive diets are often called anti-aging diets. Calorie restrictive diets build up the body faster than it can break down, thereby prolonging (rather than reducing) lifespan.

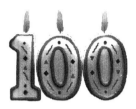

Experts Agree About The Root Cause

I covered this topic in a general manner in an earlier chapter. But, I now want to eliminate any doubt that the 100+ nutrients are indeed the answer you have been looking for to solve your health, weight, aging and longevity concerns. Here's what we know so far:

1. Doctors already know that many diseases result from nutrient deficiencies. This has been proven time and time again over the years.

2. Some very respected natural health experts and physicians over the past 80 years have figured all this out. Below are just a few of them. Feel free to Google their names if you would like more information:

   • Dr. Linus Pauling, the only man to ever win two Nobel Prizes stated: "One could trace every sickness, every disease and every ailment to a mineral deficiency! Nothing is more important than minerals to maintain a strong immune system."

- Dr. Mehmet Oz, "America's Doctor" says in an article in the January 2012 issue of *Oprah* magazine, "The number one reason Americans are heavy: the brain, very smartly, wants nutrition. But the average American is eating empty calories. So you finish that 2,000 calories and your brain says, *keep going until you get nutrients.*"

- Dr. Weston Price, a brilliant dentist, traveled the world studying third world cultures. He wondered why the most primitive people on Earth often had the most perfect bone structure, teeth and health. His only conclusion to explain these differences was their healthy diet rich in fiber, whole foods and the full spectrum of micronutrients. He documented his writings and photographs in an amazing book called *Nutrition And Physical Degeneration,* which is considered to be the Bible of natural health.

- Dr. Joel Wallach, a veterinarian and naturopath, identified the need for the spectrum of essential and trace nutrients from his work of eliminating diseases from animals and humans. He believes that everyone who dies from a natural cause ultimately dies from a nutritional deficiency. His book, *Rare Earths Forbidden Cures,* details his findings.

- Dr. Gary Todd, an eye surgeon who gave the spectrum of plant derived trace minerals to his patients, stated in a speech in Tulsa,

Oklahoma "If everyone would take two ounces of plant trace minerals each day, within a year half of the hospitals in this town would close due to a lack of patients."

• Max Gerson, M.D., creator of the famous Gerson Therapy, stated that "All people who die of natural causes die either from a nutritional deficiency or from toxicity."

• Dr. Joel Fuhrman's book *Eat To Live* is essentially all about how consuming nutrient dense, low calorie foods are the key to living a long life free of chronic disease.

• Dr. Edward Howell, father of enzymes, believed you need to first have the full spectrum of minerals in order to create optimal enzyme production, which he believed was the spark of life.

• Marie-France Muller, M.D. found that the spectrum of nutrients created the foundation necessary for the DNA to replicate cells properly and program them properly to do their job in the body.

• According to Dr. Rath, M.D.'s website, health improvements achieved with essential nutrients are so superior to conventional medical approaches for cardiovascular diseases, cancer, AIDS and other common diseases that major health insurance companies in Europe are now reimbursing the cost of these remedies (http://www4.dr-rath-foundation.org/THE FOUNDATION/ About The Dr Rath Health Foundation/ about.htm).

Please note that I could list many more similar findings. If you need more convincing please read the books in the Resources section.

3. The above mentioned experts and physicians have thousands of patients they've helped over the years to eliminate their ailments simply by changing their diet, cleansing their bodies of toxins and providing the patient with the full spectrum of nutrition. It's not complicated or rocket science. It's just common sense (but not common practice in America). You must give your body what it needs first because if you don't, it will simply break down.

4. We know that the animal feed industry adds all the nutrients each animal species needs to feed pellets. The animals eat these nutrients in every bite of their feed and rarely get sick. As experts often state, "Farmers don't have health insurance for their animals." They can't afford to have their animals get sick, so their goal is to keep them healthy as easily and inexpensively as possible. It works for animals and will work for humans as well.

    I asked our veterinarian about this recently. He's an old time country vet and has many farmers as clients. When I asked him if humans received all their nutrients each day in a pellet form like farm animals do, did he think humans could really become as disease free and healthy as animals at a minimal cost? His response? "Of course they would, but that will probably never happen because humans make too many bad choices!"

5. The oceans contain up to 84 minerals and ele-

ments and we know they once covered the entire Earth. That means these nutrients were in the soil at one time and we know they are also supposed to be in us.

6. There's nothing else it really can be, as I have shown so far in this book and in the validation-by-exclusion exercise we completed in an earlier chapter. We know everything begins at the cellular level with nutrients, DNA and enzymes. Primitive cultures from around the world simply do the basic steps and remain healthy, lean and long-lived without Western medicine or medical technology.

7. In 1912, Dr. Alexis Carrel proved that cells are basically immortal and he won a Nobel Prize for his efforts. An experiment he performed, which lasted 29 years, was to unveil something quite remarkable, something which he believed could have important significance on the life span of man in the future. Small samples of heart tissue from a chicken embryo were immersed in a solution from which they obtained all the necessary nutrients. As the cells took up the nutrient rich broth, they also excreted their metabolic wastes into the same solution. Each day the old solution was discarded and replaced with fresh nutrient broth. This chicken heart tissue lived for an astonishing 29 years, only dying when an assistant forgot to change the polluted fluid. Chickens normally live for only 7-10 years. Commenting, Dr. Carrell said: "The cell is immortal. It is merely the fluid in which it floats which degenerates. Renew this fluid at regular intervals, give the cell something on which to feed and, so far as we know, the pulsa-

tion of life may go on forever..." And, what do cells and DNA primarily feed on? You guessed it—the full spectrum 100+ essential and trace nutrients.

8. Examples of the power of minerals are everywhere in nature. Marie-France Muller points out in her book *Colloidal Minerals And Trace Elements* that when Mt. Saint Helens erupted in May 1980, the apple producers in the states of Oregon and Washington were in great despair because the thick layer of volcanic ash that covered their land completely wiped out their harvests. But, the following year, their apples grew twice as large as before and their trees bore more fruit than they ever had. The fact is that the fine powder of ash was extremely rich in trace elements which completely reinvigorated the mineral content of the soil and supercharged the apple trees.

9. Governments have been tracking the depleted mineral levels in the soil for years. If you care to see these reports and data, simply Google the appropriate terms and you will find many links.

   a. The United States government knew of the mineral depletion in our soils as early as 1936. I've put the full document, known as Senate Document 264, at the end of the book. This public document alerted Congress to the mineral depletion problem of America's soils—and the dire consequences of it—nearly 76 years ago!

   b. The U.S. Department of Agriculture published this quote in 1977: "In the future, we will not be able to rely anymore on our premise that the consumption of a varied balanced diet will provide all of the essential and trace minerals because such a diet will be very difficult to obtain for millions of people." (Nothing was done about it and the problem has only gotten worse.)

c. From the article *Vegetables Without Vitamins*, from Life Extension magazine, March 2001, below are some of the nutritional values calculated by the US Department Of Agriculture for fruits and vegetables today compared to 1975:

  i.   Apples, Vitamin A down 41%

  ii. Sweet Peppers, Vitamin C down 31%

  iii. Collard Greens, Magnesium down 85%; Potassium down 60%; Vitamin A down 45%.

  iv. Cauliflower, Vitamin B2 down 47%; Vitamin B1 down 48%; Vitamin C down 45%.

  v.   Broccoli, Vitamin A and Calcium both down 50%.

  vi. Watercress, Iron down 88%.

d. The Earth Summit was held in Rio De Janeiro in 1992. The consensus from the analytical tests concluded the soil mineral content during the last 100 years (1892 – 1992) <u>declined</u> in specific countries as follows. It was published under the World's Most Impoverished Soils (see *The Untold Truth* by Elmer Heinrich):

  i.   U.S. and Canada: an 85% reduction

  ii. South America: a 76% reduction

iii. All of Asia: a 76% reduction

iv. Europe: a 72% reduction

v. Australia: a 55% reduction.

Minerals are the "foundation of the foundation" of life. Enzymes, the catalyst of life, can't work without minerals. Vitamins can't work without minerals. Minerals are required as the spark plug that ignites virtually every chemical reaction in your body. Without minerals you would die. With fewer minerals than you need you will create aggravating symptoms, chronic conditions and diseases *before you die.*

I hope it has become obvious so far that:

- Your body needs the 100+ nutrients for every bodily function and their deficiency creates all kinds of problems and diseases for humans.

- It's difficult to obtain the full spectrum of these nutrients in adequate dosages from our foods due to the many reasons pointed out earlier.

- The deficiency of these nutrients is the most probable common sense root cause of America's health, disease and obesity problems.

- It's ridiculously easy and inexpensive to solve the problem through supplementation.

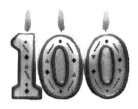

The Only Difference
You Need To Know

I by no means am a mineral expert, however the following general information will provide you with the vital basics you need to know should you choose to supplement.

Minerals exist in two forms: Non-plant based (inorganic, metallic) and plant-based (organic, non-metallic).

Non-plant based minerals are from rock, mineral salts, or clay. This is the original form of the mineral. Over time, wind and water erode rocks and rain washes the rock dust into streams, rivers, lakes and oceans. The ash from exploding volcanoes also eventually falls back to Earth and provides a good source of minerals. Flooding rivers and streams deposit the minerals in the soil and this is why land around water is typically naturally rich in minerals. According to Elmer Heinrich in his book *The Untold Truth*, inorganic minerals are said to be only five percent to eight percent absorbable by your body because they have not been "predigested" by a plant. That means they are still in their inorganic form (rock dust, clay, salt) and it's difficult for your body to absorb them. However, getting minerals in this form is certainly better than not getting any minerals at all.

Plant-based (organic) minerals, on the other hand, have been "predigested" by the plant. This means the roots of the plant absorbed the inorganic minerals from the soil and converted or predigested them into an organic form. In this form, according to Heinrich, minerals are nearly 100% absorbable and are the *same* as the minerals found in fresh fruits and vegetables. Although plants only require about nine minerals to be healthy they will take up any minerals that are in the soil and convert them to an organic plant-based form even though the plant may not need them. We eat the plant directly or its produce and we therefore ingest these plant predigested minerals that are very easy and safe for us to absorb.

The most vital difference between plant-based and non-plant based minerals is the transformation that takes place when the plant absorbs and predigests the mineral. If you consider a mineral like arsenic that is needed by your body in small quantities—in one form it's a poison yet in another form it's vital for health. How can that be? Rat poison is arsenic—inorganic arsenic. It's the raw mineral that's found in rock or salt that has not been predigested by a plant. Taken in this state, it is toxic to the body. Yet, when arsenic in the soil is taken up by the root of the plant, predigested by it (converted from inorganic to organic), and then eaten by a human or animal it poses no problems at all and is actually *required* for health. Many fruits and vegetables contain organic arsenic and aluminium and other so called "poisonous" substances. Produce like tomatoes and apples often contain organic minerals such as these. This is allowed by the FDA because it understands these minerals are safe and required by the human body in this organic (i.e. predigested) form.

Marie-France Muller, M.D. in her book *Colloidal Minerals And Trace Elements* states the following about how plant-based minerals are the preferred source by the human body:

> This does not suggest that it is a good idea for people to take excessive quantities of inorganic mineral supplements. Studies have shown that though the body will utilize a supplement in the case of a specific mineral need (such as a crisis of spasmophilia), 10 or 20 times more than the organic form of the mineral is required in order to achieve the same results. Such high dosages, however, are not easy for the body to assimilate and present the risk of an overdose that in and of itself can have adverse consequences. Ideally we should take trace elements [minerals] in the form of a complex in synergy with plant extracts in the naturally occurring form of a colloidal water of plant origin...

The safety and the absorbability factor of plant-derived minerals in a colloidal (very small) form is why my family takes plant-derived trace minerals.

Many mineral supplements boast that they are in "colloidal" or "ionic" form. This just means they are in a very small form, smaller than the size of a molecule of water and this alone is *not* a true differentiating factor among minerals. The only differentiating factor you need to be aware of is organic (plant-derived) vs. inorganic (rock, salt, or clay) forms. The organic plant-derived preferred form, as we've already discussed, is the form you want because it's been predigested by the plant, is said to be the safest, is nearly 100% absorbable by your body and is just like those found in fresh fruits and vegetables.

The food pyramid recommends we eat six or more servings of fruits and vegetables a day which is sound advice to obtain some of these nutrients. Even if you ate 100 servings of fruits and vegetables each day, experts say you would receive no more than 20 minerals in varying dosages as that's how many minerals are left in farmable soil today. As you now know, they say your body needs at least 50 more minerals than this.

For plants, humans, and animals it all starts at the same place—the minerals must be in the soil first. The plants convert these minerals into a highly absorbable organic form and humans and animals eat the plants, thereby obtaining the minerals they need. If the minerals aren't in the soil they won't be in the plants or animal products you eat. As you have learned, not only have modern farming practices depleted many of these elements from the soil, but the practice of adding pesticides to our soil further inhibits the plant's ability to absorb any minerals that do exist.

It's a double whammy. If alien visitors came to our planet after humans are extinct and learned how we abused our bodies, land and food supply in this manner, they'd scratch their head (or antenna) in confusion! They might telecommunicate to each other:

> We don't understand this species called Humans. First, they don't get the raw material nutrients their body needs in the first place to stay healthy. Then, they add pesticides to their soil that further exacer-

bates the nutrient depletion problem and also heavily pollutes their planet. Then they eat a lot of meat, which is the most inefficient source of food on their planet because it uses up precious food and fresh water supplies...and further pollutes their planet. Then they eat a lot of sugar which more rapidly depletes any nutrients they might receive. Then they load up their bodies with toxins from what they breathe, eat, drink and medicate themselves with, which further depletes nutrients in their bodies. They must have had a death wish because *they killed themselves.*

Imagine how much healthier humans and our planet would be if we took this simple, common sense, inexpensive step of giving our plants and bodies the nutrients they need to create strong immune systems in the first place. Imagine how much less pollution there would be. We'd have healthier, happier people and less pollution—it's a win-win for everyone!

In the coming chapters I'm going to begin to pull together everything that you've learned so far into practical, tangible and actionable steps.

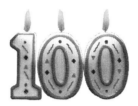

The Benefits
Happening At A Deeper
Level In Your Body

So far I've spent a lot of time writing about nutrients and the ones your body needs. Making it a top priority to get all your nutrients each day is obviously the outcome you want to achieve. However, there is a much bigger 'outcome of the outcome' that can *only* happen if you obtain all your nutrients each day. It's this deeper level of activity where *all* the horsepower resides in keeping you healthy, lean, youthful and living longer easily and inexpensively.

Here are the deeper benefits you receive when you obtain all your nutrients each day:

- The 100+ nutrients are giving your cells and DNA the full foundation of raw materials they need. Your body won't have to rob another organ, your bones or any other tissue to get the nutrients it needs or to metabolize the nutrients it's receiving. Nor will it need to rob these areas in order to neutralize toxins. *Everything is in balance.*

- The full spectrum of nutrients is allowing the full enzyme producing capacity of your body to explode into action, heal you and properly digest your foods. Optimal enzyme production is not possible without these nutrients, according to Dr. Edward Howell, the father of enzymes. Enzymes are the spark and catalyst for *everything* that happens in your body. Without enzymes life ceases to exist. It's the enzymes that burn off fat and excess calories. And it's the full spectrum of nutrients that insures your body will have the ability to make enough enzymes to do this appropriately.

- The 70+ plant based minerals in the 100+ nutrients are helping to keep your body alkaline. That's important because an alkaline solution can hold many times more oxygen than an acidic solution. That is vital because:

  - If you're acidic your body has to steal alkalizing nutrients like minerals from your organs or bones to neutralize the acidity. Some experts now believe that acidity, not the lack of calcium, may be the true root cause of osteoporosis. Your acidic body is robbing your bones of calcium and other alkalizing nutrients to neutralize your acidic condition. This is what they believe causes the bone loss and the state of osteoporosis to occur, not the lack of calcium.

  - You want to flood your body with as much oxygen as possible because according to experts most diseases, including cancer, are anaerobic (they can't survive in an oxygen rich environment). Keeping your body alkaline and oxygenated means there's a higher chance you will stop those diseases before they harm you. I've read that cancer researchers know this but have not been able to patent a man-made product to replicate this natural phenomenon. A wonderful book on the power of oxygen is by Ed McCabe called *Flood Your Body With Oxygen.* Also Google Otto Warburg, Nobel Prize winner, to learn how he cured cancers with oxygen.

- Your body is loaded with electrolytes thereby optimizing electrical communication within your body and between all cells.

- Your metabolism burns hotter with more oxygen just like a fire does. You'll burn more calories more easily, even while sleeping.

- More oxygen means less red blood cell aggregation and therefore more energy for you. You'll become more active and burn even more calories. Plus, you'll be less likely to suffer the mid-day need for coffee or sweets.

Real, *authentic energy* at the cellular level is created by the processes described above. Don't be fooled by beverages or products that claim to give you "energy" through artificial stimulation, such as caffeine or herbal extracts. Stimulants are not authentic or natural cellular energy.

Isn't it wonderful that you receive all these amazing benefits simply by receiving your complete spectrum of nutrients each day? It's such an easy and inexpensive holistic solution that it's truly astonishing.

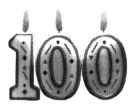

Optimizing
Cell Wall Health

Since everything begins at the cellular level it may be prudent to talk about how a cell works, in general terms. Think of each of your cells as a balloon. There's stuff on the outside, stuff on the inside and then there's a membrane that acts as the barrier between the inside and outside. The stuff on the outside (nutrients, oxygen, etc.) has to get to the inside so it has to pass through the membrane. The stuff on the inside (waste material produced from cell metabolism and toxins) needs to get to the outside so it can be expelled by the body. If the "good" stuff on the outside can't get to the inside and the "bad" stuff on the inside can't get to the outside, that's a HUGE problem.

The key to making this process work optimally is the health, flexibility and permeability of the cell wall. If this wall remains flexible like a balloon things work fine. However, if the cell becomes gummed up and stiff from a lack of nutrients or from easily oxidized fats (like cooking with vegetable oils or other unsaturated fats) or from hydrogenated fats or trans fats, that's *very* bad. Rather than resemble a ballon the cell wall more closely resembles the shell of an egg. This of course makes it much harder for the good stuff to get in and the bad stuff to get out.

Cooking with unsaturated fats causes many damaging free radicals in your body. That's why experts say you should *only* cook with saturated fats as they do not oxidize or cause free radicals. Contrary to popular belief, saturated fats are very healthy and have been used by long-lived cultures since the beginning of time. But, in America, the myth still continues that they clog your arteries and are unhealthy. This myth alone is believed to cause many health problems in America. The best book I have found on this subject is by Bruce Fife, Ph.D. and it's called *Saturated Fat May Save Your Life*.

The keys to keeping the cell wall in ideal shape are 1) get your 100+ nutrients first 2) only eat whole, natural, unprocessed fats that have never been heated or chemically processed 3) only cook with fats that are very stable and difficult to oxidize. Popular fats that meet this criteria are coconut oil, ghee, palm oil, lard and tallow.

Getting all your nutrients without optimizing the permeability of the cell wall is like waxing your car before you wash it. It's a good thing but the full synergistic effect will never be optimized.

In a later chapter you will also learn about an exercise that is excellent at keeping cells flexible and healthy.

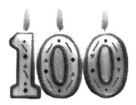

What About Fiber?

You hear a lot about the need for fiber. Fiber is a natural, indigestible carbohydrate that is found in fruits, vegetables, legumes, nuts and seeds. It is not found in oils, fats, meats or animal products. Fiber contains no nutrient value or calories. It is not something your body is asking for when you feel hunger pangs. Since fiber is indigestible and contains no calories it is often subtracted from the total carbohydrate grams for those who are trying to follow a low carbohydrate diet. The daily recommended fiber intake for an adult male is approximately 35 grams per day. For an adult female it's approximately 25 grams a day. So you know how much that is, a large orange, apple or pear may contain anywhere from three to six grams of fiber. So, if you happen to eat four apples each day you'd be getting approximately 20 grams of fiber. Nature commonly provides fiber in two to six gram "packets" in fruits and vegetables. If you happen to eat a large bowl of chili with beans you may receive up to 12 grams of fiber. Ideally, you do not want to receive all your daily fiber in one or two sittings. It's best to spread it out throughout the day as that's how nature intended it. The value of fiber in the human diet is:

- It provides "bulk" to your digestive system and helps to scrub it out and keep it clean.

- It keeps things moving along in your digestive system so toxins can't build and so bowel movements are more regular and easy.

- In your stomach, fiber can absorb liquid and make you feel full so you may eat less.

- Fiber can absorb toxins and thereby help to cleanse your body, if eaten regularly.

- Fiber may help to remove excess fat and cholesterol from the food you eat.

Please remember that your body does not ask for fiber. Fiber is something that's contained naturally in healthy food choices, almost as a by-product. Simply pumping your body full of fiber so you don't get hungry is not healthy. You can meet or exceed your daily fiber needs each day and *still* be severely nutrient deficient and prone to many diseases. Remember, you only receive your 100+ essential and trace nutrients from what you eat and drink. Fiber contains no nutrients.

Please don't fall for the hype of fiber powders, pills, potions or diet programs whose only job is to make you feel full or keep you feeling full by eating fiber. Those things may provide some value depending on your situation, but they are in no way a substitute for providing your body with the full spectrum of nutrients it needs. Losing a little weight from eating fiber does not automatically mean you're healthier or will live longer.

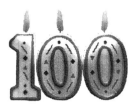

What About Digestive Health, Bowel Movements, And Gas?

Since we just talked about fiber and since fiber is often associated with "regular" bowel movements, let's talk about bowel movements.

Transit time is the time it takes something you swallow to come out in your poop. Ideal transit time is 12-18 hours. You can actually measure your transit time simply by eating corn. Few people can digest corn and therefore it's highly visible in your poop. Note the time you eat the corn and simply note the time when your poop contains the corn kernels. The elapsed time is the transit time.

The general rule is to have at minimum one bowel movement each day. Ideally you want to have two or three. Part of your bowel movement frequency depends on how much you're eating. If you eat like I suggest in this book you may only have one bowel movement a day and you will feel fine. You should also have relatively little gas. The average person passes gas about 14 times a day. Anything more than that over a period of a few days or a week could signal something is wrong. If things are working well "down there" your gas should have little to no odor.

Here are your bowel movement goals:

- Transit time should be no more than 12-18 hours.

- You should have at minimum one bowel movement per day and ideally two or three.

- It should come out easy with no need to force or strain.

- It should be firm with smooth sides yet flaky looking. That means it should hold together in the toilet bowel but when you flush it may break apart like saw dust.

- It should be light brown to medium brown in color.

- There should be very little odor if you have good transit time and if your colon is clean.

- Some experts believe it should have a nice "s curve" shape to it.

In my early thirties when my father and brother were both dying from cancer, I experienced a lot of bowel problems. I thought I was eating healthy but I felt terrible. My breakfast each day consisted of a bowl of high fiber cereal, soy milk and about one tablespoon of flax oil. At the time these items were considered healthy things to do according to the advertisements I saw on TV and in magazines. My discomfort led to a battery of medical tests including a colonoscopy to make sure there were no problems in my colon. No cause was found and it was attributed to stress (diet, not stress, was the actual problem).

In my search for a natural solution I discovered an herbal fiber product around 20 years ago that my family still takes to this day. It cleared everything up in no time and I have had no problems since. I also changed my breakfast routine and now don't use any of the products I was using then. I mention the fiber/cleansing product we use in the Resources section. My point is, just because something is heavily advertised as being healthy and good for you, it's best to listen to and trust your own body, use common sense and do your own research.

If you eat the way I suggest and you obtain all your nutrients, your bowel movements should easily meet all of the above criteria.

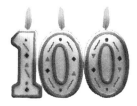

What About Sleep?

Another big problem in our society is sleep disorders that cause fatigue, low energy and a variety of other problems. Sleep disorders arise from many possible causes such as stress, anxiety, hormonal imbalances, anger, fear and of course nutrient deficiencies.

How many sleep remedies exist in America today? Tens? Hundreds? It's crazy. From a common sense standpoint, if an estimated 95% of people are not receiving their full spectrum of 100+ essential and trace nutrients each day, then most likely 95% of people aren't sleeping well. Remember, the 100+ nutrients control *everything* in your body. If you simply give your body the full spectrum of 100+ raw material nutrients it needs, your body should reward you with a sound night's sleep almost every night and plenty of authentic energy throughout the day.

If you are suffering from stress, anxiety, panic, fear, shame, worry or guilt or anything else, the 100+ nutrients will go a long way in helping to support and minimize these states. Your brain chemistry, hormone levels and how you cope and respond to stress in your life all start with nutrients—just like everything else in your body. If you're not getting all the nutrients you need, a cascade of imbalances, like dominos falling, can result in you becoming highly imbalanced and unstable. The easiest, cheapest and most common sense solution is to always get all your nutrients first.

In the Resource section at the end of the book I provide some non-nutrient solutions that work in a complementary way. Keeping with the theme throughout this book, they too are very easy, inexpensive and common sense.

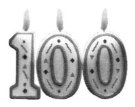

What About Cravings?

What is a craving? What causes it? Why does your body have cravings? How can you eliminate cravings?

A craving is typically defined as an intense desire for a particular thing. Cravings take many different forms. A craving for love. A craving for money. A craving for freedom. A craving for recognition. You can have a craving for virtually anything.

As it relates to nutrition, farmers have known for many years that when farm animals are mineral deficient they will exhibit signs of something called pica. Pica is just another word for craving. Pica refers to the act of the animals eating odd things like fence posts, fence hardware, water troughs, dirt and barn doors in search of minerals. If the farmer puts out a special block with minerals, the animals can lick the block to obtain the minerals they need.

Humans don't eat fence posts or the walls of their home or kitchen counters when they exhibit pica. Instead they reach for salty junk food that contains few if any nutrients and just calories. Cravings are believed to be the primary reason why Americans consume so much junk food. Our food supply is nutritionally deficient, especially in the full spectrum of minerals. And, over 90% of what Americans eat is processed! The inherent wisdom within each cell of your body knows that it needs minerals and it associates (from many generations past) a salty taste with minerals. So, you naturally crave salty foods. Experts say food manufactures know this fact and exploit it to their advantage.

Cravings primarily result from one or more of the following items:

- <u>A conditioned or learned behavioral response</u>. For example, if you condition yourself to always have a piece of chocolate after your dinner and you unexpectedly run out, you will have a craving for that chocolate because you have conditioned yourself to want it after dinner. You've created a habit.

- <u>An addiction</u>. Smokers and coffee drinkers know this all too well. You've created a conditioned or learned response and something in what you're eating, drinking, smoking or injecting is adding another "hook" to the craving. This makes it more difficult to eliminate the craving simply by stopping the habit. Your body has become dependent on a particular chemical or substance to provide a certain physical or mental sensation.

- <u>A nutritional deficiency</u>. Natural health experts say a craving primarily results from the natural wisdom of your body letting you know it needs something. Your body is raising its hand and yelling, "Hey I need this!" and giving you an *intense* desire to go find it. We've all heard of the pregnant woman who craves pickles and ice cream—a seemingly unappetizing combination. Natural health experts would say that because of the added nutritional needs of the developing baby, the mother's body is signaling intense and often strange cravings to provide the mother and her baby the nutrients they need.

Of course, cravings don't just happen to pregnant women. They happen to all of us more than we would like. Stressful situations can often trigger a craving because your body uses up its nutrient reserves to help you better cope with the stress. When all of your 100+ nutrient buckets are full and kept full every day your body has everything it needs so there is no need to crave anything. Since everything at the cellular level improves with the proper nutrients, even people who have severe drug or behavior addictions can drastically reduce or eliminate their addiction by simply supplementing with the full spectrum of nutrients, especially trace minerals.

In Dr. Joel Wallach's book *Rare Earths Forbidden Cures*, he does an excellent job of discussing, in detail, mineral deficiencies and their devastating effect on animals as well as on the physical, emotional and behavioral aspects of humans. Children in schools typically will behave much better and have greater focus when their nutrient buckets are full. A deficiency of essential and trace nutrients worsens or even causes acting-out behaviors like bullying. When all of your nutrient buckets are full you become much more balanced physically, mentally and emotionally. Your desire to overeat foods that can make you fat virtually disappears. You can still enjoy highly craved foods like potato chips, chocolate, and cake but you will be able to stop yourself when you want to. If you can't stop yourself, you know you need more trace minerals until your nutrient buckets are full. Keep your 100+ buckets full every day and you will look, feel and behave like a different person.

Drinking alcohol also rapidly depletes minerals and can cause intense cravings for more alcohol or junk food. If you have a drink every now and then you absolutely *must* obtain a regular supply of trace minerals each day. College students listen up! Your body uses up a lot of nutrients, and especially trace minerals, in the process of metabolizing alcohol. Add in the stress of studying and you see why most college students would do well to get their 100+ nutrients daily. At a minimum, they need the full spectrum of trace minerals each day. I have been told there is no better cure in the world for a hangover than to drink water several times a day that is loaded with 70+ plant-derived trace minerals. When you understand how minerals are the foundation for everything in your body, it just makes sense that this natural hangover remedy would work.

The absolute sure-fire way to stop a craving is to allow the trace minerals to pass directly over your tongue. Simply place a small amount of trace mineral powder or liquid directly on your tongue or drink eight ounces of water with one quarter teaspoon of trace mineral powder in it. The craving will disappear almost immediately.

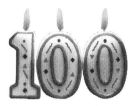

What About Weight Loss Programs?

In earlier chapters you learned the following: that approximately 85% of your weight, and how you look and feel, is determined by what you choose to put in your mouth; that 75% of the calories you burn each day is due to your Basal Metabolic Rate (BMR); how minerals fix your metabolism and alkalize your body, thereby increasing your body's ability to hold more oxygen and more oxygen makes your metabolism burn hotter; how receiving all your nutrients each day will allow you to eat normally and eliminate your desire to overeat and eliminate your cravings.

Since an estimated 95% of people are *not* getting their full spectrum of nutrients, don't you think if they did there may be little need for weight loss programs? How much easier can it get? Because people are unable to control what they put in their mouth (because they are not receiving their spectrum of nutrients each day) many industries have been created over the past 60 years to help people "compensate" for this easily solvable problem. There is a need for today's weight loss programs *only* as long as people remain confused about how to get healthy, lean, and long-lived easily and inexpensively. If people were receiving all their nutrients *first* each day and were *still* unable to control what they put in their mouth, only *then* would there be a true need for these programs.

Another issue with weight loss programs is they focus on the wrong problem. The root problem is *not* the consumption of too many calories, lack of portion control or eating the incorrect ratio of fat, protein or carbohydrates. The question that should be asked is "What's really *causing* people to eat in a way where they *desire* more calories than their body needs in the first place?" *It's not a lack of will power or self control. It's a lack of nutrients!* Remember, experts say the root cause of excess weight and obesity is a *deficiency condition of nutrients.* This creates the "symptoms" of eating too many calories and excess weight. Your body contains all the knowledge it needs to allow you to achieve and maintain your ideal weight, easily and inexpensively. You just need to give your body the raw materials it needs, *in the first place,* so it can do all of the work for you. Weight loss programs need to be focused on *nutrients first*—not calories! Solve the nutrient root cause first and the calorie problem will take care of itself *automatically!*

Let's use some common sense here and make a simple comparison of today's health beliefs to the probable health beliefs of people living 100 years ago. People from generations past seemed to stay lean relatively easily and without any special effort, pills, or potions. Was this most likely because:

- They drank eight glasses or more of water each day like we do? No. They probably only drank fluids when they were thirsty.

- They had more knowledge about health than we do today or more information about how the human body works? No.

- They went to the gym regularly and worked out incessantly? No.

- They were generally more active than we are today? Perhaps, but there were still many jobs back then which required lots of sitting, like we do today.

- They took more supplements than we do today? No, the supplement industry didn't exist then.

- They ate more whole, unprocessed foods than we do today? Yes. The prepackaged food industry was in its infancy then. People did not have as many unhealthy choices as we do today.

- They generally received more nutrients from their foods than we do today? Yes. Not only were the soils not as over-farmed, but a single orange or apple (or any other whole food for that matter) contained significantly more nutrients than today. They could eat *fewer* calories than us and still receive *more* nutrients.

Years ago, people really didn't need to try to be healthier or more fit or trim than us. They didn't have to do anything *special*. They just ate normally, rarely exercised and went about their normal daily lives. They ate more whole foods than we do and they probably received many more nutrients, water and fiber from foods than we do.

The human body today still needs the same raw materials it needed 100 years ago—or for that matter 100,000 years ago. However, today due to our modern lifestyle which is high in stress, low in nutrients and high in toxins, we need to be much more careful and work smarter to obtain the nutrients we need.

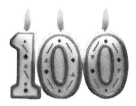

How You Can Eat Normally And Naturally— Effortlessly

How can you use all the information you've learned so far to make it easy and inexpensive to control what you put in your mouth—without feeling deprived? How can you virtually eliminate your desire to eat more calories than your body actually needs? Simple. Get all of your 100+ micronutrients each day.

Remember, you only feel hungry for two primary reasons:

1. Your body needs calories from the macronutrients protein, fat or carbohydrates
2. Your body needs micronutrients (vitamins, minerals, amino acids, essential fatty acids)

That's it. If you completely satisfy reason number two,

then the *only* reason you will experience hunger is because of reason number one. There will be *no reason* to eat more calories than your body needs. You will greatly reduce or eliminate cravings because all of your 100+ nutrient buckets will be full. If you need about 2,500 calories a day to maintain your weight—and all of your micronutrient buckets are full—there is no reason for your body to desire more than 2,500 calories a day. Your body is too smart and efficient to do that when it already has everything it needs. It's almost magical how simply getting your 100+ nutrients daily self-regulates your caloric intake and optimizes your metabolism.

Sounds too easy, right? Well, you could also say that breathing is too easy—you simply breathe in and out and magically your body knows what to do with that invisible substance you breathe in, right? If you receive all the oxygen you need there is no need for more. You breathe for only one reason—to get oxygen. Eating is a little different in that you eat for two reasons—to obtain calories and to obtain nutrients. If you're not getting your nutrients and your body keeps you hungry in search of them, you will have the unfortunate side effect of eating too many calories and gaining weight. The trick is to make sure you get all your nutrients first each day. Then, you are eating for only one reason—for calories. Since your body already has everything it needs from the nutrients, it will self-regulate its need for calories.

I hope you see that getting healthy, lean and long-lived is not confusing. It's not a mystery. Your body knows exactly what to do once you give it all the raw materials it needs. It's common sense, not rocket science. It is truly miraculous.

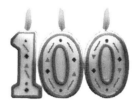

Simple Four Step Program For Success

I'm now going to start to pull together all the information you've learned up to this point. Things will get even more specific in the next chapter.

To be healthy, lean, and long-lived as easily and inexpensively as possible you need to follow only four simple steps. They are:

1. Accept personal responsibility for your own health, weight and choices
2. Cleanse (i.e. detoxify)
3. Nourish
4. Exercise (minimally)

Some people would add Hydrate as well. That's obvious and falls under the Nourish section. Drink when you are thirsty. You will also get plenty of water in the foods and beverages you consume.

Step One
"P"

"P" stands for Personal Responsibility.

There's a lot of talk today about healthcare reform in America. But what really *is* authentic healthcare reform?

Let's first cover what it *is not*:

- It *is not* about rewarding people who choose to not take care of themselves.

- It *is not* about creating new pharmaceutical preparations or medical technology that won't cure anything and will simply treat the symptoms of chronic conditions caused by improper nutrition and poor quality of life choices.

- It *is not* about making it easier or less threatening for people to make poor choices.

- It *is not* about making it easier for people to become dependent on our healthcare system.

- It *is not* about keeping people uninformed about how they can achieve their goals easily and inexpensively.

- It *is not* about doing what's good for corporate profits or the economy, but bad for citizens.

Here's what authentic healthcare reform *is* about:

- It *is* about instilling a sense of personal responsibility in people for their choices and educating them about how to make better choices.

- It *is* about teaching people how their body works and about the nutrients their body needs to remain healthy and *prevent* disease in the first place.

- It *is* about empowering people to transform—not just bombarding them with more information.

- It *is* about designing an authentic healthcare system that rewards people (with financial incentives) for staying healthy.

- It *is* about teaching people that the cure for most diseases already exists inside them and it's called their immune system. It is about teaching people how to keep their immune system healthy and robust so they can prevent diseases in the first place.

No one who takes the time or effort to take care of themselves wants to pay for those who simply choose not to. That's a bail-out and, after the financial crisis, it's very clear how those who live responsibly feel about bailing-out those who don't.

We are beyond the information age. Information is everywhere. Today, people want *transformation*—that is, to know how to find the information that really matters and *how to apply it* to transform their health and life. That's what this entire book is about.

In New Jersey where we live, no one can be denied health insurance and the premiums are the same based on gender and age. I can be a 50-year-old man who never sees a doctor, runs marathons, eats the healthiest most expensive organic diet on the planet and makes all the right choices. Yet, I pay the same insurance premium as a couch potato my age who is 200 pounds overweight, constantly sees a doctor and could care less about health and what he puts in his mouth each day! Is this a good system? No, it's a *terrible* system! Does it inspire people to take personal responsibility for their own health? No! It rewards them for doing all the wrong things—or worse yet, for doing nothing. It's like paying your top sales rep at your company, the person who brings in 80% of your sales, the same amount of money as your worst sales rep who sits around all day surfing the internet while bringing in no sales. It would never happen in the real world, but that's how it works in the healthcare world. It is not ecological. It doesn't make common sense.   And, it's *destroying* America's health.

I may never go to a doctor or hospital and my couch potato peer could go three times each week and have all kinds of tests done regularly and sure enough, my health insurance premiums go up 20% every year like clockwork just like his do. My health insurance company makes thousands of dollars of profit from my family each year while his insurance company may lose hundreds of thousands of dollars each year from him, yet our premiums go up the same each year! It's truly insane and it would be difficult to design a worse system.

Even my car insurance company rewards me for being a good driver by refunding me a portion of my premiums the longer I go without an accident. That *is* an effective incentive based system. If our government's goal is to truly reform healthcare don't you think the system should reward people for becoming healthy when they choose to invest their own time and money in their health? Of course it should.

The healthcare system is what it is. It's not directly within your control. What *is* directly within your control are your eating and lifestyle choices. Hopefully, you will become so healthy that you can literally "opt out" of America's healthcare system and only use it for true emergencies.

Step Two
"C"

"C" stands for Cleanse.

We're going to talk about two types of cleansing—physical and emotional. Each is very important.

<u>Physical Cleansing</u>

Why is there a need to physically cleanse and detoxify your body? Because each of us is loaded with toxins from medicines, personal care and hygiene products we use and from what we breathe, eat and drink. We each have between 400-800 toxins in our body at any given time, according to the article below. Additionally, an estimated 85% of us supposedly have from a few pounds up to 30 pounds of undigested food and fecal matter lodged on the walls of our intestines that's built up over our lifetime. When this debris remains in your digestive system it can create all kinds of problems.

Some of them are:

- Holding toxins in your body longer than necessary helps to create disease

- Slowing the transit time between bowel movements

- Weakening the natural peristalsis activity of your intestines that keeps the food moving through your digestive system

- Dramatically reducing nutrient absorption

- Creating cravings and imbalances as your body depletes nutrient supplies trying to neutralize the toxins

- Depleting nutrient reserves faster than necessary

- Impairing the ability of your immune system to do its job. An estimated 85% of your immune system is located in your intestines and if the walls of your intestines are coated with mucous, sludge and old fecal matter, obviously your immune system can not properly do its job.

It's no wonder some experts say "death begins in the colon."

This effect is described clearly in an article excerpt from "Most Common Toxic Materials & Their Effect in Our Body," which can be found at: http://www.testcountry. org/toxic-materials-in-our-body.htm.

Effects of Toxic Materials

The toxic materials that we are exposed to every day whether consciously or unconsciously are stored in our bodies. Studies have shown that our body stores about 400 to 800 toxic materials. They accumulate in our cells and our major organs. The major organs that are affected with these toxins are the liver, kidneys, brain and some of our glands like the adrenal and thyroid. The fertilizers in our body can be accumulated in our tissues and bones. Other substances may be stored up in the brain and thyroid gland.

Studies have further showed that a typical person, even those who live in the most remote areas in the world, has about 40 to 70 chemical residues found in their tissues.

With these unwanted toxins stored in our bodies, we may be hampered from utilizing or taking up minerals that would help us function normally. Common diseases brought about by body toxins are nutritional deficiencies, brain chemistry damages, imbalances of hormones, autoimmune deficiency, enzyme dysfunction, neurological disorder, and chronic disorders.

It is then important that we take nutritional supplements and detoxify our body every now and then. Certain therapy will also help our body to get rid of the toxins and improve our immune system and body functions for wellness.

The nonprofit Environmental Working Group analyzed the blood of newborn babies from around the country and published the results in a July 14, 2005 article titled *Body Burden – The Pollution In Newborns*. They discovered the babies contained 287 chemicals and other toxins, including 76 chemicals that cause cancer in humans and animals, 94 that are toxic to the brain and nervous system and 79 that cause birth defects and abnormal development. You can find the article on their site at www.ewg.org.

Of course, there are many more articles available about the toxins that exist in our bodies today and their damaging effects, but I think you get the point. Can you imagine starting your life on Earth today with 287 toxins and chemicals *already* in your body? It's hard to imagine. The need to cleanse your body is obviously greater now than at any other time in human history and the good news is that it's easy and inexpensive, with many available choices.

So, America is really suffering from a *dual problem* of *too few nutrients* and *too many toxins*. No wonder we're getting sicker and fatter as a country. The remaining pages will teach you how to reverse this so you will receive the proper nutrition and the fewest toxins. Experts believe these steps alone could eliminate 85% or more of America's disease, aging and obesity issues easily, inexpensively and rapidly.

Types Of Cleanses

There are two general types of cleanses—a colon cleanse and a whole body cleanse.

A colon cleanse simply cleans out the colon and often the intestines. These can take from a few days up to 30 days. The goal of a colon cleanse is to remove any old, encrusted fecal matter and mucous from the intestinal and colon walls.

A full body cleanse does the same thing as a colon cleanse *plus* it detoxifies your entire body, including your organs. It takes longer to do a whole body cleanse because you're cleansing a larger area more deeply. Depending on how you've treated your body up to this point, it may take from a few months up to a year. I am referring to a full body cleanse from this point forward as that is the only type my family has ever used.

I'm old enough to remember a time when organic food didn't exist. We simply bought fruits and vegetables, ate them and that was it. There was no discussion about whether you should buy organic or conventional fruits and vegetables. There was no need to discuss it because there was no choice. But, today it's a different world than it was thirty years ago. Today, we are bombarded with toxins from all angles and especially from our food.

Your goal to reduce the toxic load in your body is two-fold:

1. Minimize toxins entering your body
2. Maximize toxins exiting your body

Many natural health experts believe cleansing of the entire digestive tract (mouth to anus) and body (everything other than mouth to anus) is one of the single most important things you can do to improve your health. A popular natural health expert that has treated thousands of patients said in his many years of experience approximately 90% of all the diseases and health issues he witnessed simply disappeared after patients thoroughly cleansed their bodies and obtained the proper nutrition.

Remember in an earlier chapter I said that the process of digesting food is the single biggest stressor on the human body? Well, do you think it's easier for your body to digest food when your intestines and colon are clean or when they are impacted with old mucous and fecal matter? Obviously it's easier when they are clean. By not cleansing you are simply adding further stress on your digestive process and your body.

It's estimated that approximately 85% of your immune system resides in your intestines. If your intestines are caked with mucus and old fecal matter, how effective is your immune system going to be? Not very effective. I've read many times from many different sources over the years that cancer cells exist in all of us all the time. Experts say, if your immune system is functioning normally, it will identify these cancerous cells and zap them before they can do any damage. However, if your digestive system is filled with lots of gunk and toxins that are keeping your immune system from properly recognizing these cancerous cells, perhaps that's how these cells get the upper hand and begin replicating in the first place.

There are many brands of cleanses on the market. I presume they all have varying levels of effectiveness. I can only comment on the one my family has used for over 20 years and I've listed it in the Resource section. My children even used this cleanse periodically when they were young on an as-needed basis, as they still do today.

You should choose a cleanse that is right for you as there are many available at your local health food store and on the internet. Look for one that contains fiber, is all natural, non-addicting and gentle. Preferably you will buy a full body cleanse, not just a colon cleanse. You want a cleanse that you can use every day for the rest of your life, if you wish.

The general rule my family was told to follow when cleansing is this—for every year you have not cleansed you must cleanse for one week. So if you are 40 years old and have never cleansed, the rule of thumb is that it will take you 40 weeks to thoroughly cleanse. Eighty percent of the mucous and encrusted fecal matter in your digestive system may come out within the first month, but the remaining 20% may take longer to come out. Understand that virtually all tissue and organs in your body can store toxins. I was told by one cleansing expert that she had a patient whose eyes returned to their original color after she cleansed! Imagine the incredibly positive effect her cleansing had on the rest of her body, as well.

Emotional Cleansing

The same way you can have physical sludge (such as old fecal matter) clinging to your physical body and digestive tract, you can have emotional sludge (such as emotional baggage or negative programming) clinging to your mental state. This baggage can have a powerful negative effect on your mind/body connection, health and self-improvement efforts.

Every human has issues they wish to resolve and emotional baggage they wish to let go of. Everyone! I suppose it's just part of the "human condition". Some people choose to face and resolve those issues—sometimes incurring quite a bit of temporary discomfort in the process—while others go through their entire life carrying the emotional baggage that can literally make them sick. There are three things you can do with emotional baggage—express it, suppress it or let it go. The one that makes the most sense, of course, is to let it go. A therapist friend of mine believes that if people would just learn to "let it go" 98% of the world's problems would be solved.

Eckhart Tolle, the famous spiritual teacher, believes we all carry two "pain bodies" within us during our lifetime. One is the pain from your own life experiences and traumas; the other is the collective pain of all life. These are both always present and a person needs to learn how to manage them. You can read more about pain bodies in his landmark book *A New Earth.*

Ever since I read my first Wayne Dyer book called *Your Erroneous Zones* many years ago, I've been a huge fan of clearing away any emotional baggage that may be holding me back. Who wants to go through their entire life carrying around (in most cases) *someone else's* emotional baggage that happened to target you and serves absolutely no purpose except to bring you down?

Experts say that, if you're like most people, you probably grew up in a household with no shortage of negative programming, fear, depression, suffering, anxiety, shame, guilt, blame, traumas, yelling, fighting, arguing, emotional and psychological abuse, brainwashing and other dysfunctional and self-defeating circumstances. Although children may be affected differently depending on their personality or birth order, it's no wonder a mentor and coach I know said that, in his opinion, 97% of all adults have *issues*—virtually *all* of which originated in their childhood and primarily from the way they were *poorly parented*. Only about 10% of these people are brave enough to face and overcome those issues as an adult. The other 90% don't want to face the pain. He told me even though he's been helping people for many years he loses about 90% of his new patients after the first or second session. When I asked him why he said that's about how long it takes people to realize they will have to directly confront their pain, and that most people are so terrified of doing this that they quit his sessions and keep their pain suppressed.

Parents, please be aware that the effects of any dysfunction you create in (or pass to) your children as a result of you not dealing with *your own* issues, demons, negative programming, pain from your childhood or life experiences is greatly enhanced in you *and* your children if either of you is deficient in the spectrum of 100+ nutrients. Dr. Wallach in his book *Rare Earths Forbidden*

Cures discusses the effects that a lack of proper nutrition has on human behavior, brain chemistry, psychological stability and mental functioning.

If 97% of the world's problems and dysfunction are created from how we're parented, please don't be part of the 90% of people who choose not to face and correct those issues. It can be temporarily painful to face your issues but it's kind of like vomiting—it only hurts while you're doing it and you feel so much better afterwards. Your children will thank you for it, you'll become a better and stronger person who can do more good for the world and you will more closely become the person you were truly born to be. If you're interested in knowing of a few very simple and highly effective approaches to removing any emotional baggage you may have, the below low cost options don't require much money or time. You can learn about them by doing a simple internet search or by searching for them on YouTube:

- Neuro-Linguistic Programming (NLP)

- Emotional Freedom Technique (EFT), also known as Meridian Tapping

- The Sedona Method

- Self-Hypnosis by listening to CDs or MP3 sessions designed to help you overcome whatever it is you wish to overcome

- Sessions with energy healers, shamans or Reiki practitioners

The purpose of these programs is to reduce or completely eliminate the behavior, pain or "charge" around any issues you may have. I'm not a therapist but I've studied a number of these techniques and used to sell them to top executives and advertising agencies so they could better understand their target markets. I also have a number of friends who practice in these areas, so perhaps I can generally explain what the above programs do. Have you even seen a picture of a home at the ocean that is near the water's edge and is raised up on stilts? The home that is resting on the stilts is analogous to the behavior you wish to change. The stilts under the home that are holding it up are the supporting elements that allow that particular behavior to continue. The stilts represent things like beliefs, assumptions, motivations, goals, other possible choices, constraints, etc. The only way to stop the behavior is to weaken or break down enough of the supporting stilts until the home (i.e. behavior) comes crashing down. That's why it's important to use these techniques regularly–so the "stilts" don't have a chance to form in the first place. Other supplemental approaches you may consider to remove blockages include massage therapy, meditation and Reiki.

Other experts use the analogy of your childhood being like a computer hard drive. When you're born your hard drive is blank in that you have no life experience and no learned behaviors. The people who "program" your "hard drive" in your early years are your parents, siblings, aunts, uncles, etc. The majority of your programs come from your parents. So, of course, your parents program their unresolved issues, fears, demons, etc. into *your* "code". These programs act much like the programs on your computer in that they are always operating in the background, subconsciously, each and every day. When you are faced with certain life situations or choices, these programs are what silently drive your behaviors and the choices you make. When your choices bump up against reality they can begin to cause conflicts or problems. For most people, any faulty programming can exist for the majority of their adult lives unless they do the work required to reprogram their hard drive. Since most of these negative programs were created in childhood, it can be a difficult task to reprogram them unless you put forth the work. That's why you often hear about people who were in therapy for years yet showed little improvement. A therapist on TV that I happened to come across explained it this way: "Sometimes breaking away from negative childhood programming can feel like the effort required for the space shuttle to leave Earth's gravitational pull. A lot of energy may be required to "lift off" initially but the further you travel the easier it becomes to move forward faster and with much less effort." That's why it's important to experiment with different techniques to learn what works best for you.

Here's yet another more Eastern explanation that may resonate with you from a shaman I know. Each of us has our life purpose buried deep within us. It's like a bright light that is encapsulated in a tough shell that's made of layers, like the layers of an onion. Right before we're born we sign a life "contract" that lists the good and bad life experiences we *agree* to go through in life. The purpose of these experiences is to shape your soul and character into what it needs, much like the way a blacksmith hammers a shapeless piece of metal into a beautiful object. If we agree to be born we *automatically* accept this contract. From the moment we're born the hard layers around our life purpose begin to form through experiences with our parents, friends, coworkers, relatives, strangers, animals, etc. Your job, as a human, is to figure out how to crack these hard layers so you can ultimately reach and fulfill your life purpose. Some people have very thin, weak layers and understand their life purpose quickly, as that was their contract. Others have a mixture of many thick and thin layers that require more work to tunnel through. It's not better if you have thin or thick layers or many layers or just a few. What's important is that you keep working through the layers, negative programming, pain, anger, guilt, baggage (or whatever else life has dealt you) with perseverance and persistence until you reach your life purpose - that magical *force* that you care about that lights you up and creates deep passion inside you. That is the key signal that you've actually discovered your purpose. Many people simply give up the fight and just "be" for most of their lives and there's nothing wrong with that. Others scrap, struggle and wrestle any way they can to crack the layers, searching for their purpose the way a heat-seeking missile seeks its target. There's no right or wrong approach and whether you find your life purpose is not good or bad and is not related to your value as a person. However, if you discover your life purpose your "rewards" are said to be inner peace and authentic joy and fulfilment.   Pretty nice rewards!

Emotional baggage, negative programming or unresolved issues from your childhood can manifest themselves in many different ways once you become an adult. Some of them are: you become a workaholic; you become an alcoholic; you physically, mentally or emotionally abuse or bully your spouse or children; you become addicted to people, substances or behaviors; you can't stop exercising; you become obese or emaciated; you can't seem to maintain a loving or lasting relationship with a partner; you're angry and snap at people; you have issues at work or with authority; you become egotistical; you become obsessive; you become a perfectionist; you become very controlling; you have an obsession with money, success or failure; you crave power; you physically or emotionally abuse people; you're very defensive, combative or argumentative; you have phobias, etc. The list is almost endless. The key is to recognize that these issues can exist in any of us; we're all only human and no one is perfect. The issues are there for a reason; they somehow got programmed onto your "hard drive", and something is continuing to fuel them. If they exist in you, be grateful for recognizing that, and simply get them take care of.

I just read recently that the mind/body connection is so powerful, scientists now believe that your blood plate-lets become stickier when you're under stress, thereby increasing your chances of a heart attack. Addtionally, experts say that the effects of negative programming or emotional baggage can lie dormant in all of us (like a computer virus) for years. Then, if the right conditions trigger them, they can spring into action and begin their destruction. That's why they say it's so important to *regularly* cleanse and detox your thinking and emotion-al state - before any of those issues can get the best of you.

Your thoughts, emotions and stress levels are as much a part of your body as your heart, liver and lungs. It's not always easy to rid yourself of emotional baggage and negative programming, but it's certainly worth giving it a try and being persistent.

You deserve to become the authentic person, through and through, that you were meant to be in your lifetime. Everyone has issues, but if you do the work you'll reap the significant rewards. That must be why experts say that healing your own issues or ending the cycle of dys-funtion that may have been passed from your parents to you is one of the greatest gifts you can give to your-self, your partner and your children.

Step Three
"N"

"N" stands for Nourish.

There are several ways you can nourish your body to obtain the nutrients you need. They are:

1. Eating the right foods
2. Drinking the right beverages
3. Supplementing if necessary

People usually either do too much or not enough when it comes to nourishing their body. Either scenario is bad because it can create imbalances. Imbalances can lead to disease, as you know, so your goal is to always try to keep as many things in balance as possible within your body.

Remember these points as you proceed:

- 85% of your weight and how you look, feel and perform is determined by what you choose to eat and drink. You are going to learn how to nourish your body in a way that virtually elimi-nates your desire to overeat.

- 75% of the total calories you burn each day are due to your Basal Metabolic Rate (BMR) so it's vital to fix your metabolism so it burns as hot as possible.

- Your main goals when eating are to:

  - Obtain only the calories your body needs

- Obtain the micronutrients your body needs

- Do as little harm as possible to your body in the process

- Put as little stress on your digestive system as possible

- Try to make whole foods and beverages at least 80% of what you eat and drink

Next, I'll begin to categorize everything you've learned so far into general categories.

General Nourish Checklist

Below are the general daily goals you want to achieve. I provide a simpler, more concise daily checklist a few pages from here.

Every day you want to do the following:

- Get your 100+ nutrients: *Think nutrients first, taste second!* When you make a food or beverage choice I'd like you to first think about the nutrients in your choices, not taste. Ideally, you want to receive as many of your nutrients from fresh, whole food sources as possible.

- Supplement only if necessary (or for insurance): If you don't believe you can get all your nutrients from your food or if you want to be certain you obtain all your nutrients in specific dosages, then you should supplement. Supplementing is not a license to eat junk food. For instance, in my family we supplement with the 100+ nutrients even though we eat very healthy and always try to "think nutrients first" when making our food and beverage choices.

• <u>Get extra trace minerals:</u> Each morning right out of bed I try to mix 8 to 12 ounces of water with about 300 mg. of plant-derived minerals and I drink this on an empty stomach. About an hour later I have breakfast and take the 100+ nutrients (vitamins, amino acids, essential fatty acids and more trace minerals) in two separate doses—half at breakfast and half with dinner. Then at or near bedtime I take up to another 300 mg. of trace minerals with eight ounces of water. Remember, your body heals itself while you sleep. You want to make sure you have a full foundation of all the trace minerals while you sleep so healing will be maximized. It also keeps your mineral nutrient buckets full while your body heals so you don't wake up ravenous with cravings. This little step is very simple and powerful and should also help with any sleep issues you may have.

• <u>Drink enough water so you're not thirsty:</u> Most everything you drink contains water. Preferably, you want to drink natural, low calorie beverages that contain no man-made artificial sweeteners. Don't drink fruit juices or soda, or at least dramatically reduce your consumption of them. If you're a milk drinker, try to drink raw milk if it's available. I'm not sold on the eight glasses of water a day theory. It was never proven and supposedly became popularized through a statement taken out of context in a study. Many cultures around the world are healthier than Americans without drinking the amount of water we drink. Drinking more water than you need more rapidly depletes nutrient levels.

Plus, it's thought to stress your kidneys. It also dilutes stomach acid if you drink fluids with meals. This can result in undigested food and inadequate breakdown of food because the micronutrients are not fully released or absorbed.

- <u>Get fiber:</u> Fiber exists only in things that grow from the soil—fruit, vegetables, nuts, seeds, grains, and legumes. Fiber does not exist in meats or oils. Fiber fills you up, digests slowly and usually makes for more frequent and easier bowel movements. But fiber itself contains no nutrients so make sure you get your nutrients first.

- <u>Minimize toxins coming in:</u> If you can afford to eat organic food products, do so. If you can't, just wipe or wash the edible skins of fruits and vegetables with a little soap and water or produce wash. Rinse well. Eat and drink as many unprocessed products as you can. Minimize or eliminate your use of man-made sweeteners and additives.

- <u>Only eat when you are truly hungry:</u> Listen to your body. Eat at most three meals a day and only snack when you are truly hungry.

- <u>Stop eating when you are no longer hungry, not when you are full:</u> When you are no longer hungry, stop eating. By the time your brain catches up to your stomach in about 20 minutes you will feel full.

- <u>At least 80% of what you eat should be healthy, whole foods:</u> Examples include fresh fruits and vegetables, beans, nuts, seeds, whole grains, etc.

- <u>At least half of that or at least 40% of your to-</u>

tal calories should come from raw foods: Raw, fresh, whole foods (foods that have not been heated to more than 118 degrees Fahrenheit) contain all their enzymes so they help to digest themselves. This puts less stress on your digestive system. They also contain more phytonutrients and other goodies that experts say are destroyed by cooking.

- Breakfast up to lunch: Eat as much fresh fruit as you want. Sometimes I add tahini, dried coconut flakes, cinnamon, raw almonds, etc.

- Lunch up to dinner: Eat as many fresh vegetables as you want. You can eat them in a wrap, salad, hoagie roll or something similar.

- Dinner to bedtime: Eat whatever you want in moderation. Dinner can be your largest caloric meal of the day (but still comprised of healthy, whole foods) since between dinner and breakfast is the longest time you won't eat. Eating this way is in line with your natural biorhythms.

- Snack if necessary: Best choices are fresh fruit, vegetables, nuts, seeds, whole grains and water with 300 mg. of trace minerals added.

- Don't count anything: If you are getting your nutrients and doing what I recommend above you will not need to count calories or grams of fat, protein or carbohydrates. And, do not become obsessed with consuming enough protein, regardless of what you hear in the media or through advertising. Just eat a normal varied diet of fruits, vegetables, nuts, seeds and some meat, if you prefer. You will receive all the protein your body needs.

- <u>Minimize digestive stress:</u> Remember earlier I said that digestion is the largest stressor on your body? You want to eat in a way that minimizes digestive stress. If you eat the way I suggest in this section, that is, easier to digest foods for breakfast and lunch, you will automatically meet this goal. Additionally, the simple act of getting all 100+ nutrients each day will provide your body everything it needs to make digestion as easy as possible.

Below I further elaborate on some of the above points for additional clarification:

- <u>Eat only when you are truly hungry</u>. A lot of diet programs tell you to eat when you are not hungry so your body has a constant supply of fuel and so you never "pig out" from being too hungry. They suggest eating five to seven mini meals a day whether you are hungry or not. I believe your body's innate natural wisdom is far greater than what any diet guru knows. Do not override your body's innate wisdom as this goes against common sense. If you aren't hungry, don't eat. Listen to your body. If you naturally wake up at 6 a.m. but don't get hungry until 11 a.m., eat something at 11 a.m. It defies common sense to eat when you're not hungry. Your digestive system needs to rest and when you're constantly eating there is no time for it to rest. People who end up eating five to seven meals a day typically end up eating more calories as well, according to experts.

- <u>During your time of greatest activity eat the foods that are the easiest to digest</u>. What does this mean? The digestion of food is the biggest stressor on the human body, right? So, if you eat a heavy meal for breakfast, lunch or snacks, a large part of your energy is used to digest that meal. You end up feeling tired and pumping more caffeine into your body. If you eat easy-to-digest foods during your waking hours like fresh fruits and vegetables (as much as you want) you will be amazed at how much more energy you will have during the day. You also will be flooding your body with nutrients, water, fiber, enzymes, phytonutrients and nutrient cofactors. You will feel energized and amazing.

• <u>Dinner should be the largest meal of the day</u>. Again, this goes against what many popular diet books promote. But remember, we're using common sense here. We are not trying to be different or controversial. My only goal is for you to obtain the best results as easily and inexpensively as possible.

Suppose you eat dinner at 6 p.m. each evening and you wake up at 6 a.m. each morning. That's 12 hours where your body does not receive any fuel or nutrients. Since the longest span of not eating occurs for most people between dinner and morning, doesn't it make sense that your highest calorie meal should be dinner?

• I came across an article about six months ago that elaborated on the above points. The author was discussing the natural biorhythms of the human body and how, during the daytime hours, it is best to not eat heavy, high calorie foods. At around 5-6 p.m. your biorhythms change as your body naturally prepares for the evening. You should eat heavier foods and the most calories at that time. The author said this biorhythm change coincides with the fact that our longest natural period of not eating is from dinner to breakfast. Often this can be a 10-12 hour span. It makes perfect sense then that your largest caloric intake should be at dinner, to fuel your longest period between meals.

- <u>At least 80% of what you eat should be whole, unprocessed foods full of nutrients, water, fiber, healthy oils and some protein</u>. If you feel hungry and are going to eat something, your first thought should be—think nutrients first, taste second! This is the opposite of how most of the population thinks today. People get hungry and often think taste first. About 90% of what my family eats comes from the following categories. These are common items we almost always have in our home and I recommend others consider doing the same:

  - Fresh fruits (bananas, apples, pears, figs, dates, melons, grapefruit, oranges and whatever else we can find or is in season)

  - Fresh vegetables (including green leafy ones like kale, collard greens, spinach, etc.), white and sweet potatoes and virtually any other vegetables we can find

  - Coconut (usually dried flakes)

  - Dried beans and all natural canned beans (many different varieties)

  - Rice and whole grains (whole grain bread,

pasta, crackers, oatmeal and a few cereals from the health food store for the kids). Rice is usually considered to be wasted calories according to many health gurus, but in reality it's very filling, easy to digest, contains no gluten and is great with beans and fresh vegetables stirred in with it. It works—try it! Rice is also a staple food of most long-lived cultures around the world.

- Natural fats—peanut butter, tahini, ghee, real butter, olive oil, coconut oil, raw milk (or full fat organic milk if you can't find raw milk). Only choose fats that are raw and that are derived from cold pressing, expeller pressing or centrifuged (spun at high speed). NEVER eat oils processed with chemicals or heat.

- Nuts and seeds (raw when we can find them)

- Eggs (organic)

- Small quantities of meats (mostly chicken, some sliced ham and turkey for sandwiches, preferably organic; my wife is allergic to seafood/fish).

- Dairy products: Raw milk, yogurt, kefir and some cheeses, sour cream (we always choose *full fat* raw dairy products when we can). If we can't find raw dairy, we buy full fat organic dairy products. We *never* buy any "skim" dairy products, only full fat. If you're cringing at the thought of full fat dairy products, pay a visit to this site and you'll learn why: www. westonaprice.org. Most of the vital nutrients are in the fat!

- Homemade soups, stews and chili (usually with

vegetables, beans and whatever else we decide to add). Also, we add miso paste (a fermented soy product) to vegetable dips and stews.

- Condiments and spices: A good unprocessed sea salt, whole peppercorns to grind, fresh and dry onion and garlic, cayenne pepper, ketchup, mustard, jelly, most common household spices, curry, cumin, cinnamon (both ceylon and cassia), nutmeg.

- Sweeteners: Sugar, agave, molasses, raw honey, stevia, maple syrup (NO artificial sweeteners).

- Beverages: Coconut water, brewed coffee, brewed tea, water, raw milk. We're not big alcohol drinkers but when we do, it's typically dark beer or red wine. (NO fruit juices or soda.)

- Dessert-type items: Full fat organic ice cream, frozen bananas or fruit bars, dark chocolate, maybe some homemade cookies, fennel seeds (plain and candied mixed together), raw yogurt or greek yogurt.

- <u>Ideally, at least forty percent of what you eat should be raw.</u> You hear a lot today about raw foods. Eating raw scares a lot of people but if you follow the way I eat at the end of this section it is very easy. Dr. Edward Howell is known as the father of the enzyme movement. He defined a food as being raw (i.e. "live") if its enzymes are still alive. For example, when you see a banana turning brown, you think it's rotting, right? In reality what's happening is the enzymes in the banana are digesting it. Enzymes die over a temperature of about 118 degrees Fahrenheit.

That's about the same temperature where it's too hot to put food or liquids in your mouth. Could this be nature's way of alerting us as to whether a food is raw or not?

• As I discussed earlier, Dr. Howell discovered the human body produces two categories of enzymes, digestive enzymes (used to digest what you eat) and metabolic enzymes (used to repair your body). He felt these two types of enzymes were made from the same "factory." He felt this factory had a limited capacity to produce enzymes and once this supply was depleted, death would occur. His goal was to preserve the enzyme producing capacity of the body as long as possible so the patient would live as long as possible. If the patient ate "dead foods," that is, foods where all the enzymes were killed by cooking, then the body would have to make digestive enzymes to digest that "dead" food. If the body was busy making digestive enzymes this reduced its ability to make metabolic enzymes to repair the body. Eating more dead food than live food allowed the body to age more quickly because it could not be repaired in a timely manner. If this occurred long enough, a state of enzyme depletion occurred (i.e., death). The only way to keep his patients alive and healthy for as long as possible was to have them eat raw (i.e., live) foods so the foods themselves contained the enzymes necessary to digest that food. Basically, the food would digest itself "for free"—thereby taking no energy from the patient's body. In that case the body would not have to make any digestive enzymes and the entire enzyme making capacity of the body could be used to make the repairing and healing metabolic enzymes that would heal the patient. Obtaining your 100+ nutrients each day is vital in keeping your enzyme "factory" in ideal operating condition.

- This same concept was proven in a different way by a man named Francis Pottenger, who created a brilliantly simple study that measured the benefits of raw vs. dead foods consumed by cats. His famous study is known as "The Pottenger Cat Study." He was able to prove that raw, nutrient dense foods kept the cats healthy generation after generation. The cats that ate the cooked, dead foods began to show birth defects after their first litter. The easiest way to learn about his work is to simply Google "Pottenger Cat Study."

- Foods that taste great raw are:

  - All fruits

  - Most vegetables

  - Most nuts and seeds

  - Most oils and fats

  - Coconut

  - Dairy

- Fats: The prevailing belief for many years was that "fat makes you fat." Of course this was *totally wrong* but this myth still continues today because it generates billions of dollars of profits for the healthcare and processed food industries! Fats are vital and are healthy, as long as they're the right fats. Eat *only* natural, raw unprocessed fats that are cold pressed, expeller pressed or centrifuged. These processes use no high heat. NEVER eat any fats that have been extracted using high heat or chemicals. Do not eat ANY man-made or processed fats like margarine, vegetable oils, hydrogenated or trans fats. The fats we eat abundantly are real butter, ghee (clarified butter), olive oil and coconut oil. We never buy vegetable oils as they oxidize very quickly, especially when heated, due to their lack of saturated fats. This is believed to cause many harmful free radicals in the body. Experts believe this is a *major* cause of many health problems in America today. If you want to learn everything you need to know about fats, you should study Weston Price's website. It does an excellent job of clearing up any myths that exist about fats and which ones are healthy. Also, study Bruce Fife's book called *Saturated Fat May Save Your Life,* as it clears up many myths.

What about dairy? There are probably more myths about dairy products than there are about any other category. Do humans need dairy products? Is dairy healthy for humans? All I can do is tell you what my family and friends do so you can draw your own conclusions. About six years ago my family started drinking raw milk. In New Jersey where we live we can't buy raw milk, so we have to travel one hour round-trip each week to Pennsylvania to buy our weekly supply of two or three gallons. The farm we visit has raw milk, raw cheeses, raw yogurt, raw kefir, organic ice cream and many grass fed meats and free range eggs. I've never been a big milk drinker but my wife and kids enjoy it. They never get sick and are strong and healthy. My kids often comment about how many of their friends at school are sick and they seem amazed that they're not sick. They've been drinking raw milk from a young age. We've given raw milk to many people who claimed they're lactose intolerant or allergic to dairy, including my own mother. For years, these people have not been able to the drink milk commonly found in stores that has homogenized and pasteurized (i.e., it's a "dead" product in that it contains no live enzymes because it's been heated). Every one of them can drink raw milk with no problems. Actually, raw milk and cod liver oil totally stopped my mother's ulcerative colitis in only three days. Prior to this she spent about 10 years visiting doctors and trying all the popular (and expensive) pharmaceutical preparations on the market. Pretty amazing!

Like other live foods with their enzymes intact, raw milk contains all the enzymes necessary to digest itself. One of those enzymes is lactase, the enzyme responsible for digesting the lactose in milk. People who are lactose intolerant can't make the lactase enzyme so the lactose in pasteurized milk remains undigested and causes discomfort for them. With raw milk, the lactose is easily digested by the live lactase enzyme in the milk. When milk is heated through pasteurization to over 118 degrees, all the live enzymes are destroyed. It becomes a "dead" product. The lactose still remains, but the enzyme in the milk to digest it – lactase – has been destroyed from the pasteurizing. I can enthusiastically recommend only raw milk and raw dairy products as we have had nothing but success with them. You can read all about raw milk at www.realmilk.com or at the Weston Price site listed in the Resources section.

What about salt? This area, I believe, is also full of myths. Salt's reputation has been demonized but it's not fair. Real, raw salt naturally contains trace minerals but they are said to be only five to eight percent absorbable as they are in an inorganic (metallic) form. Common table salt (sodium chloride—the processed form of salt) is thought by experts to be unfriendly to your body. That's why they always recommend using a natural salt with minerals present. I've read from numerous sources that there supposedly has never been a medical study that conclusively proves salt actually causes high blood pressure. Yet, look at the billions of dollars the drug companies continue to make as long as this myth continues. Your body is electrical in nature and adequate salt intake is *absolutely required for health.* Salt insures electrical impulses work optimally in your body. In everything I've ever read, *too little salt causes many more problems than too much salt.* If you eat a high quality salt with adequate trace minerals your body recognizes it as a whole food. If you eat too much of this kind of salt your body will simply excrete what it doesn't need. However, when you eat salt without minerals (like common table salt), it's believed two things happen: *First,* your body views it as a "poison", tries to dilute it by pulling water out of your tissue and places that water in your bloodstream in an effort to "flush" the poison out. This added volume of water in your bloodstream naturally creates more pressure on the arteries thereby creating what is diagnosed as high blood pressure. You're then given drugs called diuretics, whose only job is to *force* water out of your bloodstream thereby reducing the volume of water in your arteries to relieve the "high" pressure. So, what is helping you and protecting you (the additional water that your very wise body moved into your bloodstream to protect you) is now being *artificially* forced out because of Western medicine's misunderstanding of what's *really* happening. *Second,* the common table salt crystals may actually "scratch" the inside of your arteries, thereby causing them to bleed.

Cholesterol (the good guy) rushes to those damaged areas to seal the arteries to stop the bleeding. Cholesterol is incriminated as the "bad guy" when actually it saved your life. That's why my family ONLY uses a good quality, natural sea salt that contains many trace minerals. We also use an iodized sea salt periodically to make sure our thyroid gland is nourished properly from the iodine. Because people have been brainwashed that salt is evil and they've reduced their salt intake dramatically, the lack of iodine (from salt) in our diets has now become a whole new problem in America. Forget about all the nonsene and simply use a good quality salt with all its trace minerals intact and salt your food as you like.

What about snacking? Snacking is fine as long as you're experiencing true hunger. Drink a glass of water with 300 mg. of plant minerals dissolved in it first and wait 15 minutes to make sure you're truly hungry, and not simply thirsty. Great snacks are:

- Fresh fruit

- Fresh vegetables with a humus or yogurt dip, or in a wrap

- Nuts or seeds

- Beans (all natural flavored beans in a can are fine but we usually wash off the sauce first)

- Whole grain bread with a pat of butter or peanut butter

What about cholesterol? Apparently it's been known for years that eating high cholesterol foods does not significantly increase cholesterol levels in your body, cause heart disease or cause cholesterol build-up on your arteries. But just recently on TV I heard a news reporter talking about how to lower cholesterol! You probably don't realize that about 80% of the cholesterol in your body is made by your liver, so the cholesterol from your diet has little impact. Also, nearly half of the people who die from heart disease have below normal cholesterol levels. And, many people who have very high cholesterol are perfectly healthy with no cardiovascular problems at all. Cholesterol is also required for adequate hormonal and brain health and is the true "good guy" in your body in many ways. It rushes to the rescue when your body is damaged. It doesn't just start depositing itself on your arterial walls because there is *too much of it*. There's most likely damage in those areas (caused by your faulty diet and poor lifestyle choices) and cholesterol is showing up there to *save your life*. To never worry about your cholesterol levels again, please visit Dr. Weston Price's website or purchase a book by Dr. Bruce Fife called *Saturated Fat May Save Your Life*. My family does not pay any attention to our cholesterol levels. We take our 100+ nutrients so everything in our body remains in balance, we follow the advice in this book, eat healthy, natural whole foods and trust our body to sort everything else out.

What about cooking methods? We rarely use a microwave oven and instead use a steamer, traditional stove top or oven. If you've ever done the popular test at home where you try to sprout a bean seed using room temperature water that was initially heated using a microwave oven, you'll understand why we rarely use one. The seed rots instead of sprouting! The only oils we cook with are saturated oils like coconut oil and ghee, as any others can burn and oxidize thereby creating many free radicals. Some experts believe that cooking with oils that oxidize easily (like most mono and polyunsaturated oils) is a leading cause of why cholesterol in your blood is "forced" onto the walls of your arteries - to repair the arterial damage caused by the free radicals. Other saturated fat oils you can cook with are lard and tallow (yes, these are healthy!). Butter is ok too, but it can burn quite easily due to its unsaturated fat content.

As I discussed earlier, the goals of nourishing your body are simply to:

- First, obtain all the nutrients your body needs

- Second, obtain the calories your body needs

- Third, *do as little harm and add as little stress as possible* to your body in the process

If you follow my suggestions in this section you will achieve all of those goals, easily and inexpensively.

Step Four
"E"

"E" stands for Exercise.

In an earlier chapter I mentioned that health experts believe approximately 85% of the way you look, feel and perform is determined by your diet. Only about 15% is determined by everything else, including exercise.

The primary goals of exercise, in no particular order, are to:

- Strengthen your body

- Stretch your body

- Keep your joints limber and lubricated

- Oxygenate your body

- Strengthen your cardiovascular system

- Increase your circulation

- Promote the circulation of lymphatic fluid (which has no pump and only circulates via gravity)

- Reduce stress and clear your thinking

- Keep your metabolism high (this will happen naturally as muscle builds and fat recedes)

- Enhance cell wall flexibility and permeability

- Do nothing to damage or tear down your body

The sole purpose of exercise should not be to 'burn off' the extra calories you consume from poor eating habits.

What's the best exercise that will do all of the above in the shortest period of time? According to experts, it's rebounding. Rebounding is the practice of jumping on a mini indoor trampoline—which is referred to as a rebounder. Rebounders are typically three or four feet in diameter and can be used in almost any room in your home. I recall reading articles where NASA said that rebounding is the most perfect exercise a human can do because it meets all of the above criteria. What sold me on rebounding was the common sense of it. I am exercising every single cell in my body at the same moment. The creator of one of the rebounders my family uses said in one of his promotional videos: "When you do a bicep curl you are exercising just the bicep and some surrounding tissue. But, what about the rest of your body? What if you could do a bicep curl on all 100 trillion cells in your body at the same time?" Sold!

When you rebound you tone every inch of your body and every cell in your body at the same time. In today's time-crazed world, I can't think of any exercise that provides greater return on your time investment.

At a minimum, I try to rebound for 10 minutes a day six days a week. If I'm in the mood, I might do other exercises as well. Rebounding meets all the goals of exercise listed above. Plus, it dramatically increases your balance and is fun.

A few very unique additional benefits of rebounding that you may not know about are also very impressive:

- Eliminate cellulite: I've read stories and testimonials of women who ate right, exercised regularly and were already thin yet still could not lose stubborn cellulite on their legs and buttocks. After only a few weeks on a rebounder the cellulite disappeared.

- Face-lift: If you stretch your neck and chin upwards as you're rebounding it will tighten any loose skin on your neck and face. If you make funny faces while rebounding you supposedly will obtain the closest thing to a face-lift that you can achieve, without surgery.

Rebounders can be purchased at a sporting goods store for under $100. You can also find better ones on the internet costing up to $1,000. I went through a few of the lower cost versions (the straps tore) until I settled on the brands I use now that cost a few hundred dollars and are of superior quality. I mention these brands in the Resources section.

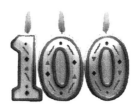

Your Daily Checklist

The one-page checklist a few pages from here summarizes everything you've learned in this book. Please consider placing it in multiple locations in your home and workplace, as a reminder.

The overall theme of the checklist is *common sense, easy, inexpensive* and *natural*. The big-picture goals are:

1. Nourish your body first with the full spectrum of 100+ nutrients it needs to work optimally in every area and eliminate any imbalances that may exist. You will *minimize* calories by *maximizing* nutrition. You can add the nutrients, especially the trace minerals to soups, beverages (water, tea, coffee, smoothies, etc.), cereal, etc. This will do two key things:

    a. It will fill your nutrient "buckets" and allow you to control the amount of food you put in your mouth so you can eat naturally.

    b. It will rebalance all the functions of your

body so they work optimally as they were designed to do.

Remember, the <u>first step</u> to resolving <u>any</u> of your health, weight, wellness, aging, behavior or addiction issues should <u>always</u> be to get your 100+ nutrients <u>first</u>, to nourish and rebalance your body.

2. You're going to eat naturally and only when you're truly hungry. You will eat only whole, natural foods, beverages and fats. You don't need to buy any commercial meal replacement products, energy drinks, powders or shots, or participate in any type of weight-loss program, unless you choose to. Minimize or drastically reduce your use of fruit juices, soda and artificial sweeteners.

3. You're not going to count calories or worry about grams or ratios of protein, carbohydrates or fats.

4. You will automatically receive adequate fiber, water, protein, phytonutrients, enzymes, antioxidants and electrolytes.

5. You will alkalize and highly oxygenate your body, automatically.

6. You will obtain some minimal movement or exercise. You may do more if you wish.

7. You will physically and emotional cleanse your body on an as-needed basis.

8. You may make adjustments to the steps or shuffle things around to fit your personal habits and lifestyle—just make sure you do the steps.

If you follow the steps on the next page you should effectively be able to opt-out of America's healthcare system, except for emergency situations.

From the book: *Lean And Healthy To 100*

1. Accept personal responsibility for your health, weight and choices.

2. Nourish: Get Your 100+ Nutrients:
   a. At minimum each day, get 70 or more plant trace minerals (approximately 600 mg. for every 100 pounds of body weight) from supplements.
   b. Ideally, also obtain the remaining 31 essential nutrients: 16 vitamins, 12 amino acids, 3 EFAs from food or supplements.

3. Cleanse
   a. Physically cleanse to remove toxins inside your body.
   b. Have at minimum one bowel movement each day.
   c. Emotionally cleanse to remove toxic emotional baggage.

4. Drink healthy fluids: Natural, low calorie fluids; virtually no soda or fruit juices.

5. Eat: Always THINK NUTRIENTS FIRST, taste second.
   a. Eat only when hungry: Drink water with some trace minerals in it and wait 15 minutes to verify hunger.
   b. Stop eating when no longer hungry, not full.
   c. Get 80% or more of total calories from whole, natural, unprocessed foods and at least half of those calories from raw (unheated) foods.
   d. Get fiber: About 35 grams for a man and 25 grams for a woman.
   e. Minimize physical toxins coming in: Eat organic foods if possible; no man-made chemicals, preservatives, fats or artificial sweeteners.
   f. Eat up to three meals a day (only when hungry):
      i. Breakfast up to lunch: Eat mostly fresh fruit, as much as you want.
      ii. Lunch up to dinner: Eat mostly fresh vegetables, as much as you want.
      iii. Dinner to bedtime: Eat what you want in moderation. This can be your largest caloric meal of the day, preferably of whole foods. Don't splurge.
   g. Snack (if truly hungry): Best choices: fresh fruits, vegetables, nuts, seeds, whole grains, raw dairy. Test hunger first by drinking water with trace minerals and waiting 15 minutes.
   h. Eat only natural fats and oils from expeller, cold pressing or centrifuge extraction; eat no hydrogenated or trans fats, vegetable oils or margarine.
   i. Don't count anything: Eat naturally, simply listen to and trust your body.
   j. Minimize digestive stress: See point "5c" above; eat raw dairy or a little fermented miso paste for added intestinal health.
   k. Enjoy a special treat if you wish: Up to 10%-15% of daily calories and preferably made of whole, real, natural foods; nothing man-made or artificial.
   l. Cooking: No microwaves; only heat coconut oil, ghee, palm oil, lard or tallow.

6. Exercise: Rebound at least 10 minutes. Do additional exercising if you'd like.

7. Miscellaneous: Sleep six to eight hours/night; if you drink alcohol, follow current guidelines; only use natural, unprocessed sea salt.

HOW MANY OF THESE STEPS DID YOU DO TODAY?
www.adviceformychildren.com

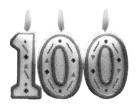

A Typical Day For Me

Below is a typical day of eating for me. Remember, you only eat for two *biological* reasons - nutrients and calories. When you get all your 100+ nutrients first and keep your nutrient buckets full you will naturally eat less and remain satisfied. Americans today do the opposite - too many calories and too few nutrients. That's why they eat more calories than they need to and have so many health issues. Getting your nutrients first also changes your internal biochemistry so unhealthy "trigger" foods and cravings don't sabotage your ability to control what you put in your body.

- Wake up and mix up to 300 mg. trace minerals in about 8 oz of water and drink on an empty stomach. (November through March I also add 1/2 tablespoon of green barley powder for additional support to avoid getting a cold.)

- Do some stretching, then rebound for 10 minutes.

- Breakfast: Most often fresh fruit (couple of apples plus whole banana plus coconut flakes plus some nuts plus cinnamon and maybe a little tahini and high nutrient salt). Other times, two eggs sunny side up (to preserve the nutrients in the yolks), piece of whole grain toast (may add bacon on occasion). Always sip a heavily diluted iced coffee with about 100 mg trace mineral powder mixed in and usually a teaspoon of very dark chocolate powder.

- Take the first half-dose of all 100+ nutrients after breakfast.

- Usually go to the bathroom after breakfast.

- Lunch: Usually fresh or roasted vegetables (in a salad or a wrap or a hollowed out hoagie roll). Sometimes soup or chili or even a slice of veggie pizza, but always whole, natural foods. Usually drink an iced beverage like fresh brewed tea or water with fresh lemon.

- Around 3-4 p.m., if I'm hungry, perhaps a snack of another 300 mg of trace minerals in water and maybe a handful of raw nuts or a piece of fruit, or both.

- Dinner: We vary our dinners but it's mainly comprised of cooked whole, natural foods (e.g. meat, beans, veggies, potatoes, soup, rice, salad, pasta, fruit, etc.) Dessert: If we eat it, which is not that often, it's most always made of whole, natural foods.

- After dinner, take second half-dose of 100+ nutrients.

- Sometime between dinner and bedtime I'll usually drink a glass of water with up to another 300 mg of trace minerals and possibly have a light snack.

- Usually go to the bathroom again between dinner and bedtime.

- Go to bed. If I happen to be doing a physical internal cleanse I'll take that right at bedtime. If I have any emotional baggage bothering me I'll take care of that at bedtime, as well.

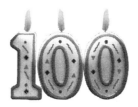

What Food And Beverage Manufacturers And Restaurants Can Do To Help

Experts estimate that, unbelievably, over 90% of food consumed by Americans is processed. That means vitamins, minerals, amino acids, essential fatty acids, enzymes, antioxidants, electrolytes, phytonutrients and nutrient cofactors—all the things your body needs to be healthy, lean and long-lived—are either removed from that food or greatly diminished compared to their fresh, whole food equivalents. In most cases, all you obtain from processed foods are calories and little to no nutrients. And as you now know that's called empty calories and it keeps you hungry and makes you gain weight easily.

I don't know how the CEO's of some of these companies can sleep at night knowing the kinds of products their company makes and thinking they're doing something positive for the world. The only way I can reconcile it in my own mind is to think "if consumers didn't buy these products they *would go away.*" But, American citizens— the ones complaining about skyrocketing healthcare premiums, increasing waistlines and health issues—*are* the ones buying these products. Consumers are keeping these companies in business and are ultimately to blame for the success of these companies.

However, there *are* food and beverage manufacturers, restaurants, coffee shops and fast-food chains that *are* interested in providing healthier products they can truly be proud of—and they are always looking for the next big thing in their category. They have to create new products that consumers want to buy and that the competition doesn't have.

If you saw two competing brands of cookies on the grocery store shelf and one boasted that it contained the full spectrum of 100+ essential and trace nutrients or the spectrum of 70+ plant-derived trace minerals—and was only slightly more costly than another brand that didn't contain them—which brand would you buy for your children? All things being equal you'd buy the brand with the higher nutrient content, right?

I'm certain the next big thing in the food, beverage, and restaurant industries will be to fortify virtually all foods and beverages with, at a minimum, the full spectrum of 70+ plant derived minerals. I believe this will be bigger than the organic movement once consumers realize that receiving the full spectrum of trace minerals each day provides far greater benefits to their health than simply eating organic products. For the manufacturer, it differentiates them from the competition while not really changing any of their manufacturing processes. It's just another ingredient—a comparatively inexpensive ingredient at that. For the consumer it does not change taste. It only adds benefits and increases their brand loyalty. Manufacturers could even boast that their foods are nutrient dense and support weight loss! It's certainly not a license to gorge yourself on these foods but if you do enjoy them periodically, you'd know you're receiving a wide spectrum of nutrients as well.

Imagine how this idea would help food and beverage companies, restaurants, fast-food chains, coffee shops and consumers. What if your favorite coffee chain offered your Mocha Java Caramel Frappuccino with a shot of 70+ minerals? It's a win for companies, a win for consumers and a win for our country's health! The idea of companies adding these vital nutrients to their products could make a huge positive impact on the health of Americans. Remember, you vote with your wallet. You should only buy what you'd be proud to serve your own family or manufacture yourself.

Side note: Several years ago as I began to understand the power of these nutrients I hired a beverage laboratory to professionally create what I called Earth's Ultimate Enhanced Hydration^{sm}. I thought this was a great way to get the word out to the world about the power of these nutrients. I was certain my formula would eliminate some of the top competitors in the industry as it contains all the nutrients mentioned in this book, plus antioxidants and electrolytes. It also tastes great, is all natural and contains less than 10 calories a serving. Little did I know the amount of capital that was required to successfully break into the beverage space! The formula is complete if any company out there is interested in adopting it as their own. It could be on store shelves within 30 days and would really do adults, children, athletes, students and the military a world of good! The formula took about three years to develop and to complete taste-testing with various age groups, until we got it just right.

If you like the idea of corporations adding these nutrients to their products, you can write directly to the CEO's of these companies. Tell them the kinds of products you are interested in having them create and the kinds of nutrients you'd like to see added to those products. Remember, you—the American consumer—controls the sales of every company. Companies can't force you to buy their products. You only buy what you consciously choose to buy. So, tell them what you want. Vote with your wallet. There's a very good chance you'll get what you want. It will be better for their business, you and your family's health and our country.

Here is the link to the list of the largest food and beverage companies in America for 2011, in case you wish to write to their top executives to suggest they fortify their foods with the nutrients outlined in this book: http://www.foodprocessing.com/top100/index.html.

If you click on any company name in the list its mailing address will appear at the top left of the page. In the first paragraph it provides the CEO's name.

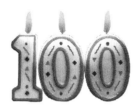

Write To The President About How To Fix America's Healthcare Problems

After reading this book you know more about how to become lean, healthy and long-lived than most people on the planet. So, why not put your newfound knowledge to good use?

You've seen how and why an estimated 95% of people are missing the basic raw materials to keep their body healthy, lean, and long-lived easily and inexpensively. Now that you know how easy it is to achieve these three goals simultaneously, you certainly don't want to keep paying skyrocketing health insurance premiums, do you? I mean, if a family of four can spend no more than $1,000 per year to obtain all the nutrients in the EAT Nutrients Pyramid—nutrients that are the absolute foundation of health, leanness, and longevity—why would you want to continue to pay $15,000 each year in health insurance premiums if you're lean and healthy? Wouldn't you like to receive a refund of $7,000 or more per year as a reward for not getting sick? I sure would.

The current battle in Washington to provide all Americans with health insurance may be morally correct but will do nothing to solve the root cause of America's health and obesity problems. Providing all citizens with health insurance does nothing to move our country even one step closer to curing cancer, heart disease, strokes, diabetes or any other disease. Most health experts would agree that virtually all ailments and diseases are already curable and even totally preventable by following steps such as those outlined in this book.

The only true, honest and humane health reform is if our government actively educates all citizens about the topics and remedies in books like this one. The government should also make sure that our food supply meets minimal levels of nutrition before any product is allowed to be sold to the American public—minimum levels of vitamins, trace minerals, amino acids and essential fatty acids. Soils should also be monitored.

Think of all the money employers would save if their employees were sick fewer days. If you never get sick and your colleagues are sick often, you're saving the company money and they're costing the company money. Shouldn't you get a bonus for not being sick? Think about how much companies—with tens, hundreds or thousands of employees—spend on sick days and lost productivity each year. If corporations taught their employees the principles in this book so the employees could become healthier, wouldn't that give the company a lot of leverage to lower its health insurance premiums? Shouldn't the employees who aren't getting sick share in that savings? It makes sense since they're putting forth effort to save the company money while also being present and productive at work more often. If I owned a large company, I might even consider buying the nutrients for my employees or at least reimbursing my employees who bought the nutrients as a perk or benefit (a billionaire in Las Vegas did something similar for his thousands of employees, and this supposedly is already being done by Europe's healthcare system). After all, if my employees are sick less, are more productive, healthier and more emotionally stable and focused at work because they're getting the full spectrum of nutrition their body needs, that certainly benefits me immensely as their employer - whether I save anything on overall health insurance premiums or not.

All of these ideas reward people for staying healthy. It moves us closer to a preventative, incentive based healthcare system which is what America really needs. As Albert Einstein said "You can't solve problems with the same level of thinking that created them." *The only way to fix America's healthcare crisis is to make people healthier.* And the absolute first thing you do when you want to make someone healthier is to make sure they get the foundation of 100+ essential and trace nutrients their body needs.

Think of how a health insurance company makes the most profit—by continuing to receive insurance premiums (revenue) and minimizing the amount they have to pay out in healthcare expenses for its members. If I was the CEO of a health insurance company and revenue from my premiums remained the same but I had to pay out 50% less in service costs because my members were healthier, I'd be jumping with joy. I would look like a genius and my shareholders would love me. I would look even more like a genius if I decided to reward my members, who were responsible for my savings, with a partial refund of their annual insurance premiums. My company or shareholders would keep the other portion of the savings. It's a win-win for everyone.

This is a true preventative, incentive based model. All the savings are generated simply by educating and encouraging people to *first* get the nutrients their body needs every day. Healthier choices will naturally follow as cravings disappear, people have less pain, more energy, are sleeping better, etc. No one has a problem with this model in the world of car insurance, why shouldn't the same model apply to health insurance?

You can write directly to our President about these and other ideas you may have by going to this website: http://www.whitehouse.gov/contact. You can complete the contact form or mail a letter. Supposedly he tries to read up to 1,500 letters a month. Maybe yours will be one of them. I've written a few times already and I hope you will too.

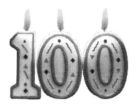

Keeping Your Money Healthy And Long-Lived, Too

I want to touch on this point briefly since you're most likely going to be living a lot longer if you do what's suggested in this book. You therefore want to make sure your money, savings, or nest egg survives at least as long as you do.

A few years ago, once I became confident that I understood the areas of health, leanness, and longevity, my next area of focus became how to make sure our savings would also last.

For 25 years I've been a passionate student of the stock market, but with today's new world *disorder* in the financial markets, it's gotten a lot tougher to protect your money, let alone to make money. Today, you can literally lose half or more of your life savings in just a few months. Through my years of investment research, I've come across a few methods of protecting and growing our nest-egg that seem to work very well, even in the new world disorder that began in 2008 when the housing bubble burst.

On my website, there is a navigation tab relating to financial health. This page generally describes what I've done in this area and eludes to some upcoming special reports I will be publishing on how you can protect your money and even achieve a historic average annual return greater than the world's greatest investor—Warren Buffett.

If you're interested in learning more about this area and staying up-to-date on when these reports will be ready, please enter your email address on the homepage. When these reports are ready, I will alert you.

A short while ago I mentioned to an acquaintance of mine, who is older than me, about this book. She wanted to know what the book was about. After I told her she sighed and said "I won't be buying it." I was shocked and asked her why. She said "Because, I don't want to live that long!" I told her she could remain in great health if she followed the checklist. She replied "Well, I guess I would buy it, but I don't have enough money to live that long."

So, she *did* want to live to 100 in good health if she could, *and* if her money lasted that long. I told her to visit our website so she could learn how to do both! Again, it's much easier than you think, but you have to follow the checklist I developed that will appear in an upcoming report. Please register so you don't miss it.

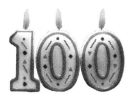

What Congress Knew That We Didn't

This document was authored by Dr. Charles Northen. It is his plea to Congress in 1936 that America's soils are heavily depleted of minerals, and that it is true cause for alarm for the health of our citizens and country.

This *public document* was presented to Congress by Mr. Fletcher June 1, 1936 and ordered to be printed by the United States Government Printing Office in 1936 during The 74th Congress, Second Session, Document No. 264. Unfortunately, Congress did nothing after this plea.

This is the unedited, original version of this document. Dr. Northen goes into detail about the problems that result in people, animals and plants when minerals and trace minerals are no longer present in the soil. It's quite lengthy, but also highly impactful. You will learn that much of what natural health experts are saying today was true *over 75 years ago*! The problems detailed in this letter have only gotten much worse since then.

Protect your health by reading this document and by getting your nutrients first each day. Remember, the below document was presented to Congress in *1936!*

*****

Do you know that most of us today are suffering from certain dangerous diet deficiencies which cannot be remedied until the depleted soils from which our foods come are brought into proper mineral balance?

The alarming fact is that foods—fruit and vegetables and grains—now being raised on millions of acres of land no longer contain enough of certain needed minerals, are starving us—no matter how much of them we eat! This talk about minerals is novel and quite startling. In fact, a realization of the importance of minerals in food is so new that the textbooks on nutritional dietetics contain very little about it. Nevertheless it is something that concerns all of us, and the further we delve into it the more startling it becomes.

You'd think, wouldn't you, that a carrot is a carrot—that one is about as good as another as far as nourishment is concerned? But it isn't; one carrot may look and taste like another and yet be lacking in the particular mineral element which our system requires and which carrots are supposed to contain. Laboratory tests prove that the fruits, the vegetables, the grains, the eggs and even the milk and the meats of today are not what they were a few generations ago. (Which doubtless explains why our forefathers [and fore mothers] thrived on a selection of foods that would starve us!) No one of today can eat enough fruits and vegetables to supply their system with the mineral salts they require for perfect health, because their stomach isn't big enough to hold them! And we are running to big stomachs. No longer does a balanced and fully nourishing diet consist merely of so many calories or certain vitamins or a fixed proportion of starches, proteins, and carbohydrates. We now know that it must contain, in addition, something like a score of mineral salts.

It is bad news to learn from our leading authorities that 99 percent of the American people are deficient in these minerals, and that a marked deficiency in any one of the more important minerals actually results in disease. Any upset of the balance, any considerable lack of one or another element, however microscopic the body requirement may be, and we sicken, suffer, shorten our lives. This discovery is one of the latest and most important contributions of science to the problem of human health. So far as the records go, the first man in this field of research, the first to demonstrate that most human foods of our day are poor in minerals and that their proportions are not balanced, was Dr. Charles Northen an Alabama physician now living in Orlando, Florida. His discoveries and achievements are of enormous importance to mankind. Following a wide experience in general practice, Dr. Northen specialized in stomach diseases and nutritional disorder. Later, he moved to New York and made extensive studies along this line, in conjunction with a famous French scientist from Sorbonne. In the course of that work he convinced himself that there was little authentic, definite information on the chemistry of foods, and that no dependence could be placed on existing data. He asked himself how foods could be used intelligently in the treatment of disease, when they differed so widely in content. The answer seemed to be that they could not be used intelligently.

In establishing the fact that serious deficiencies existed and in searching out the reasons therefore, he made an extensive study of the soil. It was he who first voiced the surprising assertion that we must make soil building the basis of food building in order to accomplish human building. "Bear in mind," says Dr. Northen, "that minerals are vital to human metabolism and health—and that no plant or animal can appropriate to itself any mineral which is not present in the soil upon which it feeds.

"When I first made this statement I was ridiculed, for up to that time people had paid little attention to food deficiencies and even less to soil deficiencies. Men eminent in medicine denied there was any such thing as vegetables and fruits that did not contain sufficient minerals for human needs. Eminent agricultural authorities insisted that all soil contained all necessary minerals. They reasoned that plants take what they need, and that it is the function of the human body to appropriate what it requires. Failure to do so, they said, was a symptom of disorder. "Some of our respected authorities even claimed that the so-called secondary minerals played no part whatever in human health. It is only recently that such men as Dr. McCollum of Johns Hopkins, Dr. Mendel of Yale, Dr. Sherman of Columbia, Dr. Lipman of Rutgers, and Drs. H.G. Knight and Oswald Schreiner of the United States Department of Agriculture have agreed that these minerals are essential to plant, animal, and human feeding. "We know that vitamins are complex substances which are indispensable to nutrition, and that each of them is of importance for the normal function of some special structure in the body. Disorder and disease result from any vitamin deficiency. "It is not commonly realized, however, that vitamins control the body's appropriation of minerals, and in the absence of minerals they have no function to perform. Lacking vitamins, the system can make some use of minerals, but lacking minerals, vitamins are useless. "Neither does the layman realize that there may be a pronounced difference in both foods and soils—to them one vegetable, one glass of milk, or one egg is about the same as another. Dirt is dirt, too, and they assume that by adding a little fertilizer to it, a satisfactory vegetable or fruit can be grown.

"The truth is that our foods vary enormously in value, and some of them aren't worth eating, as food. For example, vegetation grown in one part of the country may assay 1,100 parts, per billion, of iodine, as against 20 in that grown elsewhere. Processed milk has run anywhere from 362 parts, per million, of iodine and 127 of iron, down to nothing.

"Some of our lands, even unhappily for us, have been systematically robbing the poor soils and the good soils alike of the very substances most necessary to health, growth, long life, and resistance to disease. Up to the time I began experimenting, almost nothing had been done to make good the theft. "The more I studied nutritional problems and the effects of mineral deficiencies upon disease, the more plainly I saw that here lay the most direct approach to better health, and the more important it became in my mind to find a method of restoring those missing minerals to our foods. "The subject interested me so profoundly that I retired from active medical practice and for a good many years now I have devoted myself to it. It's a fascinating subject, for it goes to the heart of human betterment."

The results obtained by Dr. Northen are outstanding. By putting back into foods the stuff that foods are made of, he has proved himself to be a real miracle man of medicine, for he has opened up the shortest and most rational route to better health. He showed first that it should be done, and then that it could be done. He doubled and redoubled the natural mineral content of fruits and vegetables. He improved the quality of milk by increasing the iron and the iodine in it. He caused hens to lay eggs richer in the vital elements. By scientific soil feeding, he raised better seed potatoes in Maine, better grapes in California, Better oranges in Florida, and better field crops in other States. (By "better" is meant not only an improvement in food value but also an increase in quantity and quality.)

Before going further into the results he has obtained, let's see just what is involved in this matter of "mineral deficiencies," what it may mean to our health, and how it may affect the growth and development, both mental and physical, of our children. We know that rats, guinea pigs, and other animals can be fed into a diseased condition and out again by controlling only the minerals in their food. A 10-year test with rats proved that by withholding calcium they can be bred down to a third of the size of those fed with an adequate amount of that mineral. Their intelligence, too, can be controlled by mineral feeding as readily as can their size, their bony structure, and their general health.

Place a number of these little animals inside a maze after starving some of them in a certain mineral element. The starved ones will be unable to find their way out, whereas the others will have little or no difficulty in getting out. Their dispositions can be altered by mineral feeding. They can be made quarrelsome and belligerent; they can even be turned into cannibals and be made to devour each other. A cage full of normal rats will live in amity. Restrict their calcium, and they will become irritable and draw apart from one another. Then they will begin to fight. Restore their calcium balance and they will grow more friendly; in time they will begin to sleep in a pile as before.

Many backward children are "stupid" merely because they are deficient in magnesia. We punish them for OUR failure to feed them properly. Certainly our physical wellbeing is more directly dependent upon the minerals we take into our systems than upon the calories or vitamins or upon the precise proportions of starch, protein, or carbohydrates we consume. It is now agreed that at least 16 mineral elements are indispensable for normal nutrition, and several more are always found in small amounts in the body, although their precise physiological role has not been determined. Of the 11 indispensable salts, calcium, phosphorous, and iron are perhaps the most important.

Calcium is the dominant nerve controller; it powerfully affects the cell formation of all living things and regulates nerve action. It governs contractibility of the muscles and the rhythmic beat of the heart. It also coordinates the other mineral elements and corrects disturbances made by them. It works only in sunlight. Vitamin D is its buddy.

Dr. Sherman of Columbia asserts that 50 percent of the American people are starving for calcium. A recent article in the *Journal of the American Medical Association* stated that out of 4,000 cases in New York Hospital, only two were not suffering from a lack of calcium. What does such a deficiency mean? How would it affect your health or mine? So many morbid conditions and actual diseases may result that it is almost hopeless to catalog them. Included in the list are rickets, bony deformities, bad teeth, nervous disorders, reduced resistance to other diseases, fatigability, and behavior disturbances such as incorrigibility, assaultiveness, non-adaptability.

Here's one specific example: The soil around a certain Midwest city is poor in calcium. Three hundred children of this community were examined and nearly 90 percent had bad teeth, 69 percent showed affections of the nose and throat, swollen glands, enlarged or diseased tonsils. More than one-third had defective vision, round shoulders, bow legs, and anemia. Calcium and phosphorous appear to pull in double harness. A child requires as much per day as two grown men, but studies indicate a common deficiency of both in our food. Research on farm animals point to a deficiency of one or the other as the cause of serious losses to the farmers, and when the soil is poor in phosphorous, these animals become bone-chewers. Dr. McCollum says that when there are enough phosphates in the blood there can be no dental decay. Iron is an essential constituent of the oxygen-carrying pigment of the blood: iron starvation results in anaemia, and yet iron cannot be assimilated unless some copper is contained in the diet. In Florida many cattle die from an obscure disease called "salt sickness." It has been found to arise from a lack of iron and copper in the soil and hence in the grass. A man may starve for want of these elements just as a beef "critter" starves. If Iodine is not present in our foods the function of the thyroid gland is disturbed and goiter afflicts us. The human body requires only fourteen-thousandths of a milligram daily, yet we have a distinct "goiter belt" in the Great Lakes section, and in parts of the Northwest the soil is so poor in iodine that the disease is common.

So it goes, down through the list, each mineral element playing a definite role in nutrition. A characteristic set of symptoms, just as specific as any vitamin-deficiency disease, follows a deficiency in any one of them. It is alarming, therefore, to face the fact that we are starving for these precious, health-giving substances. Very well, you say, if our foods are poor in the mineral salts they are supposed to contain, why not resort to dosing?

That is precisely what is being done, or attempted. However, those who should know assert that the human system cannot appropriate those elements to the best advantage in any but the food form. At best, only a part of them in the form of drugs can be utilized by the body, and certain dieticians go so far as to say it is a waste of effort to fool with them. Calcium, for instance, cannot be supplied in any form of medication with lasting effect. But there is a more potent reason why the curing of diet deficiencies by drugging hasn't worked out so well. Consider those 16 indispensable elements and those others which presumably perform some obscure function as yet undetermined. Aside from calcium and phosphorous, they are needed only in infinitesimal quantities, and the activity of one may be dependent upon the presence of another. To determine the precise requirements of each individual case and to attempt to weigh it out on a druggist's scale would appear hopeless.

It is a problem and a serious one. But here is the hopeful side of the picture: Nature can and will solve it if she is encouraged to do so. The minerals in fruit and vegetables are colloidal; i.e. they are in a state of such extremely fine suspension that they can be assimilated by the human system: It is merely a question of giving back to nature the materials with which she works. We must rebuild our soils: Put back the minerals we have taken out. That sounds difficult but it isn't. Neither is it expensive. Therein lies the short cut to better health and longer life.

When Dr. Northen first asserted that many foods were lacking in mineral content and that this deficiency was due solely to an absence of those elements in the soil, his findings were challenged and he was called a crank. But differences of opinion in the medical profession are not uncommon—it was only 60 years ago that the Medical Society of Boston passed a resolution condemning the use of bathtubs—and he persisted in his assertions that inasmuch as foods did not contain what they were supposed to contain, no physician could with certainty prescribe a diet to overcome physical ills.

He showed that the textbooks are not dependable because many of the analyses in them were made many years ago, perhaps from products raised in virgin soils, whereas our soils have been constantly depleted. Soil analysis, he pointed out, reflect only the content of samples. One analysis may be entirely different from another made 10 miles away. "And so what?" came the query. Dr. Northen undertook to demonstrate that something could be done about it. By reestablishing a proper soil balance he actually grew crops that contained an ample amount of desired minerals. This was incredible. It was contrary to the books and it upset everything connected with diet practice. The scoffers began to pay attention to him. Recently the Southern Medical Association, realizing the hopelessness of trying to remedy nutritional deficiencies without positive factors to work with, recommended a careful study to determine the real mineral content of foodstuffs and the variations due to soil depletion in different localities. These progressive medical men are awake to the importance of prevention.

Dr. Northen went even further and proved that crops

grown in a properly mineralized soil were bigger and better; that seeds germinated quicker, grew more rapidly and made larger plants; that trees were healthier and put on more fruit of better quality.

By increasing the mineral content of citrus fruit he likewise improved its texture, its appearance and its flavor. He experimented with a variety of growing things, and in every case the story was the same. By mineralizing the feed at poultry farms, he got more and better eggs; by balancing pasture soils, he produced richer milk. Persistently he hammered home to farmers, to doctors, and to the general public the thought that life depends upon the minerals. His work led him into a careful study of the effects of climate, sunlight, ultraviolet and thermal rays upon plant, animal, and human hygiene. In consequence he moved to Florida. People familiar with his work consider him the most valuable man in the State. I met him by reason of the fact that I was harassed by certain soil problems on my Florida farm which had baffled the best chemists and fertilizer experts available.

He is an elderly, retiring man, with a warm smile and an engaging personality. He is a trifle shy until he opens up on his pet topic; then his diffidence disappears and he speaks with authority. His mind is a storehouse crammed with precise, scientific data about soil, and food chemistry, the complicated life processes of plants, animals, and human beings—and the effect of malnutrition upon all three. He is perhaps as close to the secret of life as any man anywhere. "Do you call yourself a soil or a food chemist?" I inquired.

"Neither. I'm an M.D. My work lies in the field of biochemistry and nutrition. I gave up medicine because this is a wider and more important work. Sick soils mean sick plants, sick animals, and sick people. Physical, mental, and moral fitness depends largely upon an ample supply and a proper proportion of the minerals in our foods. Nerve function, nerve stability, nerve-cell-building likewise depend thereon. I'm really a doctor of sick soils."

"Do you mean to imply that the vegetables I'm raising on my farm are sick?" I asked. "Precisely! They're as weak and undernourished as anaemic children. They're not much good as food. Look at the pests and the disease that plague them. Insecticides cost farmers nearly as much as fertilizers these days. A healthy plant, however, grown in soil properly balanced, can and will resist most insect pests. That very characteristic makes it a better food product. You have tuberculosis and pneumonia germ in your system but you're strong enough to throw them off. Similarly, a really healthy plant will pretty nearly take care of itself in the battle against insects and blights—and will also give the human system what it requires." "Good heavens! Do you realize what that means to agriculture?" "Perfectly. Enormous saving. Better crops. Lowered living costs to the rest of us. But I'm not so much interested in agriculture as in health." "It sounds beautifully theoretical and utterly impractical to me," I told the doctor, whereupon he gave me some of his case records.

For instance, in an orange grove infested with scale, when he restored the mineral balance to part of the soil, the trees growing in that part became clean while the rest remained diseased. By the same means he had grown healthy rosebushes between rows that were riddled by insects. He had grown tomato and cucumber plants, both healthy and diseased, where the vines intertwined. The bugs ate up the diseased and refused to touch the healthy plants! He showed me interesting analysis of citrus fruit, the chemistry and the food value of which accurately reflected the soil treatment the trees had received.

There is no space here to go fully into Dr. Northen's work but it is of such importance as to rank with that of Burbank, the plant wizard, and with that of our famous physiologists and nutritional experts. "Healthy plants mean healthy people", said he. "We can't raise a strong race on a weak soil. Why don't you try mending the deficiencies on your farm and growing more minerals into your crops?" I did try and I succeeded. I was planting a large acreage of celery and under Dr. Northen's direction I fed minerals into certain blocks of the land in varying amounts. When the plants from this soil were mature I had them analysed, along with celery from other parts of the State. It was the most careful and comprehensive study of the kind ever made, and it included over 250 separate chemical determinations. I was amazed to learn that my celery had more than twice the mineral content of the best grown elsewhere. Furthermore, it kept much better, with and without refrigeration, proving that the cell structure was sounder.

In 1927, Mr. W. W. Kincaid, a "gentleman farmer" of Niagara Falls, heard an address by Dr. Northen and was so impressed that he began extensive experiments in the mineral feeding of plants and animals. The results he has accomplished are conspicuous. He set himself the task of increasing the iodine in the milk from his dairy herd. He has succeeded in adding both iodine and iron so liberally that one glass of his milk contains all of these minerals that an adult person requires for a day.

Is this significant? Listen to these incredible figures taken from a bulletin of the South Carolina Food Research Commission: "In many sections three out of five persons have goiter and a recent estimate states that 30 million people in the United States suffer from it." Foods rich in iodine are of the greatest importance to these sufferers. Mr. Kincaid took a brown Swiss heifer calf which was dropped in the stockyards, and by raising her on mineralized pasturage and a properly balanced diet made her the third all-time champion of her breed! In one season she gave 21,924 pounds of milk. He raised her butterfat production from 410 pounds in one year to 1,037 pounds. Results like these are of incalculable importance.

Others besides Mr. Kincaid are following the trail Dr. Northen blazed. Similar experiments with milk have been made in Illinois and nearly every fertilizer company is beginning to urge use of the rare mineral elements. As an example I quote from statements of a subsidiary of one of the leading copper companies: Many States show a marked reduction in the productive capacity of the soil in many districts amounting to a 25 to 50 percent reduction in the last 50 years. Some areas show a tenfold variation in calcium. Some show a sixtyfold variation in phosphorus. Authorities see soil depletion, barren livestock, increased human death rate due to heart disease, deformities, arthritis, increased dental caries, all due to lack of essential minerals in plant food. "It is neither a complicated nor an expensive undertaking to restore our soils to balance and thereby work a real miracle in the control of disease," says Dr. Northen. "As a matter of fact, it's a money-making move for the farmer, and any competent soil chemist can tell them how to proceed. "First determine by analysis the precise chemistry of any given soil, then correct the deficiencies by putting down enough of the missing elements to restore its balance. The same care should be used as in prescribing for a sick patient, for proportions are of vital importance. "In my early experiments I found it extremely difficult to get the variety of minerals needed in the form in which I wanted to use them but advancement in chemistry, and especially our ever-increasing knowledge of colloidal chemistry, has solved that difficulty. It is now possible, by use of minerals in colloidal form, to prescribe a cheap and effective system of soil correction which meets this vital need and one which fits in admirably with nature's plans. "Soils seriously deficient in minerals cannot produce plant life competent to maintain our needs, and with the continuous cropping and shipping away of those concentrates, the condition becomes worse. "A famous nutrition authority recently said, 'One sure way to end the American people's susceptibility to infection is to supply through food a balanced ration of iron, copper, and other metals. An organism supplied with a diet adequate to, or preferably in excess of, all mineral requirements may so utilize these elements as to produce artificially by our present method of immunization. You can't make up the deficiency by using patent medicine.' "He's absolutely right. Prevention of disease is easier, more practical, and more economical than cure, but not until foods are standardized on a basis of what they contain instead of what they look like can the dietician prescribe them with intelligence and with effect. "There was a time when medical therapy had no standards because the therapeutic elements in drugs had not been definitely determined on a chemical basis. Pharmaceutical houses have changed all that. Food chemistry, on the other hand, has depended almost entirely upon governmental agencies for its research, and in our real knowledge of values we are about where medicine was a century ago.

"Disease preys most surely and most viciously on the undernourishment and unfit plants, animals, and human beings alike, and when the importance of these obscure mineral elements is fully realized the chemistry of life will have to be rewritten. No one knows their mental or bodily capacity, how well they can feel or how long they can live, for we are all cripples and weaklings. It is a disgrace to science. Happily, that chemistry is being rewritten and we are on our way to better health by returning to the soil the things we have stolen from it. "The public can help; it can hasten the change. How? By demanding quality in its food. By insisting that our doctors and our health departments establish scientific standards of nutritional value. "The growers will quickly respond. They can put back those minerals almost overnight, and by doing so they can actually make money through bigger and better crops. "It is simpler to cure sick soils than sick people—which shall we choose?"

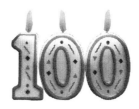

Resources

For the most current information please visit our website at www.adviceformychildren.com.

Products We Use

- Please visit our website for the most current, updated list.

Websites
(a few popular ones)

- Weston Price, DDS www.westonaprice.org

- Dr. Joseph Mercola, M.D. www.mercola.com

- Kaiser Family Foundation, www.kff.org

- About Raw Dairy, www.realmilk.com

Letting Go Of Emotional Baggage
(please visit our website for additional direct links)

- The Sedona Method, http://tinyurl.com/sedona100

- Meridian Tapping (EFT), www.thetappingsolution.com or visit www.youtube.com and enter EFT or Emotional Freedom Technique in the search bar

- Self Hypnosis, visit www.youtube.com for techniques to investigate

- For NLP, visit www.youtube.com for techniques to investigate

- For energy healers or to learn about Reiki visit www.youtube.com

Books
(these will get you started; visit our website for direct links)

- *Nutrition And Physical Degeneration,* Dr. Weston Price

- *Blue Zones,* Dan Buettner

- *Rare Earths Forbidden Cures,* Dr. Joel D. Wallach & Ma Lan, M.D.

- *Immortality,* Dr. Joel Wallach & Dr. Ma Lan, M.D.

- *Eat To Live,* Joel Fuhrman, M.D.

- *The Enzyme Factor,* Hiromi Shinya, M.D.

- *Enzyme Nutrition,* Dr. Edward Howell

- *Food Enzymes For Health & Longevity,* Dr. Edward Howell

- *The Untold Truth,* Elmer Heinrich

- *The Root Of All Disease,* Elmer Heinrich

- *Nutrition, Health & Disease,* Gary Price Todd, M.D.

- *Acquiring Optimal Health,* Gary Price Todd, M.D.

- *Eat Fat Look Thin*, Bruce Fife, N.D.

- *Saturated Fat May Save Your Life,* Bruce Fife, N.D.

- *Know Your Fats: The Complete Primer For Understanding The Nutrition Of Fats, Oils And Cholesterol,* Mary G. Enig, Ph.D.

- *Fats are Good for You and Other Secrets: How Saturated Fat And Cholesterol Actually Benefit The Body,* Jon J. Kabara, Ph.D.

- *Colloidal Minerals And Trace Elements,* Marie-France Muller, M.D.

Index

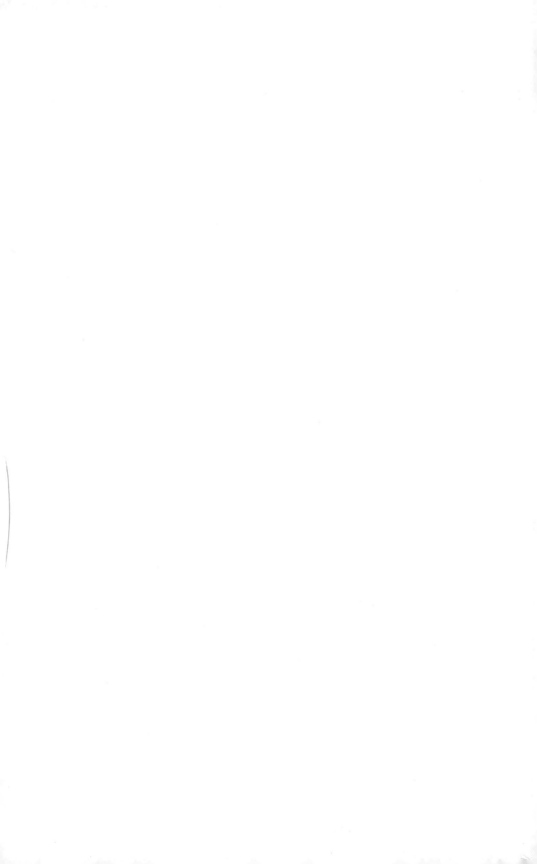